Yoania Hernández Arguelles
Greta Madruga García
Marilyn Contreras Tristá

# Chronic periodontal disease and osteoarticular diseases

Yoania Hernández Arguelles
Greta Madruga García
Marilyn Contreras Tristá

# Chronic periodontal disease and osteoarticular diseases

## Behavior in the Elderly

ScienciaScripts

**Imprint**



Cover image: www.ingimage.com

This book is a translation from the original published under ISBN 978-613-9-44153-2.

Publisher:
Sciencia Scripts
is a trademark of
Dodo Books Indian Ocean Ltd. and OmniScriptum S.R.L publishing group

120 High Road, East Finchley, London, N2 9ED, United Kingdom
Str. Armeneasca 28/1, office 1, Chisinau MD-2012, Republic of Moldova, Europe
Printed at: see last page
**ISBN: 978-620-8-22975-7**

**Title:**

# Chronic Periodontal Disease and Osteoarticular Disease Behaviour in Older Adults

**Authors:**

Dr. Yoania Hernández Arguelles.

First Degree Specialist in General Comprehensive Stomatology
Dr. Greta Madruga García.

First Degree Specialist in General Comprehensive Stomatology. Assistant Professor

Lic. Marilyn Contreras Tristá

Degree in Stomatological Care. Assistant Professor

**2024**

## Summary

**Introduction:** Chronic periodontal disease presents a strong relationship with systemic diseases, going deeper into this contributes to improve the quality of life of patients. **General objective: to** describe the relationship between chronic periodontal disease and osteoarticular diseases in older adult patients. **Methodology:** A cross-sectional descriptive observational study was carried out. The research took place in the Stomatological Service of the Nguyen Van Troi Polyclinic from January 2023 to May 2024. The population consisted of all patients with osteoarticular diseases rheumatoid arthritis and osteoporosis and chronic periodontal disease, aged 51-70 years, who gave their informed consent to participate in the study. The sample was obtained by simple random sampling and consisted of 32 patients. The following variables were used: age, sex, clinical signs of chronic periodontal disease, bone loss, tooth mobility, real pockets, risk factors, chronic periodontal disease and osteoarticular diseases.

**Results:** In our study it was observed that the age group most affected by osteoarticular and periodontal diseases was 61- 65 years and the sex most affected was female.

**Conclusions:** The relationship between osteoarticular diseases and the presence of chronic periodontal disease was evidenced.

**Key words:** osteoarticular diseases, chronic periodontal disease, relationship.

## Table of contents:

## Introduction

In recent years, with the advancement and updating of dentistry and the importance of collaboration with other medical branches, it has been possible to study the effects of systemic diseases at the oral level. It is now known that periodontitis has an influence on the pathogenesis of certain systemic diseases, and that it can increase the risk of presenting them, which has given rise to the appearance and development of Periodontal Medicine. [1]

Severe periodontal disease, which affects the tissues surrounding and supporting the tooth, is the sixth most commonly encountered disease worldwide with an overall prevalence of 11.2% and affects around 743 million people. [2, 3,4]

The prevalence of periodontal disease in Latin America was as follows: Gingivitis: Ecuador 22.4%, Cuba 16.7%, Peru 49.4%, Argentina 60%, Uruguay 44%, Venezuela 26.6%, Brazil 74%, Mexico 45%, Chile 32.6%. In the case of Periodontitis: Ecuador 1.9%, Cuba 36.1%, Peru 17.3%, Argentina 26.4%, Uruguay 16%, Venezuela 15.67%, Brazil 15.3%, Mexico 18%, Chile 30.1%.[5, 6]

In Cuba, periodontal diseases occupy the second place among oral health problems, they are present from childhood, increase in incidence with age and constitute the main cause of dental loss after the age of 35. They also cause aesthetic, anatomical and functional changes that affect the integrity of those affected. In economic terms, periodontopathies cause individual and collective affectations, as well as a significant expenditure of human and material resources. [7,8]

Osteoarticular diseases comprise more than 150 disorders affecting the locomotor system. These pathologies rank fourth in morbidity among the elderly and account for 10 % of reported conditions, after ophthalmological diseases, diseases of the mouth and teeth.[9, 10]

On the impact and prevalence of rheumatic diseases, the Spanish Society of Rheumatology estimates that worldwide this pathology affects between 0.5 and 0.8 % of the population, approximately 1710 million people worldwide have musculoskeletal disorders, i.e. approximately five people per thousand worldwide. High-income countries are the most affected in terms of number of people: 441 million, followed by countries in the Western Pacific Region with 427 million, and the South-East Asia Region with 369 million.[11,12]

In the case of rheumatoid arthritis, it is more frequent in women, with a ratio of 3 women for every man with a 3:1 ratio. An overall prevalence of rheumatoid arthritis was recently estimated at 0.46% with a 95% confidence interval of 0.390.54.[13, 14,15]

While osteoporosis affects about 75 million people in Europe, the United States and Japan. The prevalence of the disease is approximately 21% of women between 50 and 84 years of age.[16]

In Cuba the prevalence of osteoporosis is 10-30 % in postmenopausal women and 6-10 % in men over 50 years of age depending on whether bone mass is measured at one or more sites. With 18% of the nearly 12 million Cubans aged 60 and over, it is to be expected that osteoporosis will be identified as a health problem for Cubans. The most ageing provinces in the country are Villa Clara and Havana, with a rate of 17.4% and 17.1% respectively, so it is worth noting that our province is a potential for the prevalence of these diseases.[11, 17,18]

Stomatologists and physicians should join forces for the comprehensive management of patients with rheumatic diseases who present with some degree of periodontal disease, which will allow for better therapeutic options and contribute to improving quality of life. [19]

The stomatologist, in particular, can evaluate and treat the periodontal condition of patients with these pathologies at an early stage, which places him or her in the first line of prevention. In our province, studies have been carried out on this subject that have shown the possible relationship between periodontal disease and osteoarticular diseases, however, in the health area corresponding to the Nguyen Van Troi Polyclinic in Cascajal, there are no previous studies on this subject. In addition, a high number of patients with osteoarticular diseases were found to have chronic periodontal disease, and further research is needed.

**Scientific problem:**

Is there a relationship between osteoarticular diseases and the occurrence of chronic periodontal disease in older adult dental patients attending the Nguyen Van Troi Dental Clinic from January 2023 to May 2024?

**Objectives:**

**General Objective:**

To describe the relationship between chronic periodontal disease and the osteoarticular diseases rheumatoid arthritis and osteoporosis in the older adult patient.

**Specific Objectives:**

1. Describe the sample according to age and sex.
2. Characterise pathologies according to clinical variables of interest.
3. Determine common risk factors for osteoarticular diseases and chronic periodontal disease.
4. To establish the relationship between osteoarticular diseases and chronic periodontal disease in the older adult patient.

## Theoretical framework:

For the World Health Organisation (WHO), oral health goes beyond having healthy teeth; the WHO emphasises that oral health is an essential part of general health for people's well-being, and implies being free from chronic orofacial pain, cancer of the mouth and pharynx, alterations in the soft tissues of the mouth: tongue, gums and oral mucosa, congenital defects such as lesions and fissures of the lip and/or palate, and other diseases that affect the craniofacial complex. Other more comprehensive approaches such as Brazilian collective health, with the help of social sciences, contribute additional elements to the definition of oral health, understood as: A set of objective conditions: biological and subjective: psychological, which enable human beings to carry out functions such as chewing, swallowing, phonation; also due to the aesthetic dimension inherent to the anatomical region, to exercise adequate self-esteem and to relate socially without inhibitions. These conditions must correspond to an absence of active disease at levels that enable the individual to perform the aforementioned functions adequately and allow him/her to feel well, thus contributing to his/her general health. [20]

There are a number of criteria proposed to determine whether a condition can be considered a public health problem, these are: the distribution and extent of the condition; severe consequences in terms of social, psychological and economic impacts on individuals, communities and health services; whether it generates a considerable economic cost to individuals and society; and whether there are effective methods available to prevent, cure and alleviate the disease. These criteria are fully met in the case of periodontal disease. Consequently, oral disease represents, in terms of the WHO, a major public health challenge deriving its importance mainly from the overall burden of disease, the costs related to its treatment, oral pathology being considered the fourth most costly to treat, and the possibility of applying effective preventive measures.[7]

For the World Health Organisation, periodontal disease is a public health problem in industrialised countries and increasingly in the developing world, affecting the quality of life of those who suffer from it. The most common periodontal disease is chronic immunoinflammatory disease. [15, 21, 22, 23]

### Periodontal disease

Periodontal disease is one of the most common diseases that the dental professional may encounter in the oral cavity, are multifactorial in origin and linked to modifiable and non-modifiable risk factors. Periodontal disease is caused by the accumulation of microorganisms around the tooth with the stimulation of the immune system activating a massive innate and adaptive immune response.[24, 25] There are about 800 species of bacteria in the oral cavity and there is a complex interaction between bacterial infection and host response. They constitute a group of disorders of the periodontium, mostly of infectious origin that cause progressive destruction of the tooth-supporting apparatus: loss of the periodontal ligament, bone destruction, formation of periodontal pockets, gingival recessions and tooth loss. [26, 27,28]

Its most common type over the years has been chronic immuno-inflammatory disease.

Aetiology and pathogenesis of chronic periodontal disease:

The increase in bacterial surface molecules, such as lipopolysaccharides, stimulates the synthesis of cytokines and inflammatory mediators, which in turn promote the release of matrix metalloproteinases. These tissue enzymes are involved in extracellular matrix remodelling and bone destruction. Recent studies have proven that these deleterious effects are not only limited to the oral cavity, but affect the body as a whole. [25]

The inflammatory process begins with the migration of phagocytes to the site of injury by neutrophils and macrophages. This process is promoted, at least in part, by the gingival epithelium releasing chemical mediators such as interleukins, prostaglandin E2 and tumour necrosis factor alpha, which recruit neutrophils.[7]

The presence of pro-inflammatory cytokines from periodontal tissues are responsible for gingival inflammation. When the acute inflammatory response is insufficient, these cytokines stimulate hepatocytes to secrete acute phase proteins, such as C-reactive protein during the chronic systemic inflammatory process, which is a biomarker of non-specific inflammation.[29]

These phagocytic cells express specific receptors on their plasma membrane that recognise and bind to surface molecules on bacteria, such as Toll-like receptors. Similarly, proteins of the plasma complement system make pathogens more susceptible to the action of these phagocytes. This initial response eliminates microbes, followed by efficient clearance of necrotic tissue cellular detritus and apoptotic neutrophils by mononuclear cells, such as monocytes and macrophages. [7]

With an efficient immune system no damage occurs around the tooth and bacteria are removed. However, when bacteria continue to proliferate or if the immune response is deficient, acute periodontal inflammation becomes chronic and additional mediators are released. These events recruit more immune cells, such as T-cells and monocytes. The prolonged inflammatory process then induces resorption of alveolar bone by osteoclasts and degradation of ligament fibres by matrix metalloproteinases, as well as the formation of granulation tissue.[7, 25]

Biofilm formation:

Biofilm formation can be divided into three phases: formation of a film on the tooth surface, initial or primary colonisation and secondary colonisation and maturation of the plaque. As a final result, the mature Dentobacterial Plaque is formed. [7]

Species mostly associated with chronic gingivitis:

Gram positive: Streptococcus sanguis, Streptococcus mitis, Streptococcus intermedius, Streptococcus Oralis and Gram negative: Fusobacterium Nucleatum, Prevotella intermedia,

Species of: Haemophilus, Capnocytophaga and Campylobacter.[7]

Species mostly associated with chronic periodontitis: high concentrations of spirochetes and anaerobic and Gram-negative species: Agregatibacter Actinomycetencomitans, Prevotella intermedia, Eikenella corrodens, Fusobacterium Nucleatum, Treponema species and Eubacterium. [7]

Initial injury:

It is characterised by accumulation of bacterial plaque, dental plaque increases blood flow, gaps between endothelial cells and capillaries, outflow of crevicular fluid into saliva, migration of polymorphonuclears by adhesion molecules, lymphocytes are retained and then lost.[30]

Early phase:

It is characterised by plaque accumulation in week 1, vasodilatation below the junctional epithelium, leukocyte infiltrate: lymphocytes and polymorphonuclear, inflammatory infiltrate 15% of connective tissue in volume, collagen destruction necessary for tissue displacement: spacing process, detectable inflammatory changes: week 2.[30]

Established injury:

This stage is clinically characterised by obvious gingival changes in shape, colour, surface texture and haemorrhagic tendency, leading to the diagnosis of chronic, moderate or severe gingivitis. Microscopically, an intense chronic inflammatory reaction can be seen, with a predominance of plasmacytes in the infiltrate. There is increased collagen destruction which is reflected in the formation of periodontal pockets.[30]

Advanced injury:

In this lesion, there is evidence of increased pocket depth, apical migration of the junctional epithelium, apical descent of bacterial plaque, microbial multiplication in an anaerobic ecological niche, loss of alveolar bone, loss of gingival and periodontal fibres, plasma cells are the most abundant cell type in this lesion.[30]

Risk factors for chronic periodontal disease:

Nowadays and after numerous epidemiological studies, the idea of the existence of certain risk factors that modulate the susceptibility or resistance of the host to suffer periodontal disease is accepted, therefore, several causes are involved in its development. Diagnosis and identification of risk factors are essential to establish an adequate treatment plan. The association of local, functional and systemic aetiological factors with periodontal diseases can vary at different times during a person's life. It follows that the timely identification of such factors is essential to reduce the current state of the disease, prevent its onset and halt its progression, a necessary condition to determine its onset, progression and extent.[31]

Five risk factors for chronic immuno-inflammatory periodontopathies are now well documented:

The microbiota of the furrow.

Smoking.

Diabetes mellitus.

Stress.

The genetic factor.[7]

The analysis of the effects of risk factors on periodontal disease is complex, because of the incidence over a long period of time of several factors, which may include confounding variables. Moreover, the risk factor-disease association is not necessarily a cause-effect association, i.e. causal and non-causal relationships may exist.[32]

Microbiota of the gingival sulcus:

The biofilm is of highly organised bacterial origin in a favourable ecological niche for its growth and development, which with the help of additional factors of local and systemic origin causes contamination and destruction of the supporting tissues of the tooth epithelium, connective tissue, periodontal ligament, alveolar bone and root cementum. When periodontal lesions occur, the normal microbiota mutates into a pathogenic microbiota with a significant increase of Porphyromona gingivalis. As the microbiota mutates, there is an interaction with the individual's defences, and it is at this stage that inflammation and periodontal disease occur. [20, 29, 33,34]

Smoking:

The negative effects on periodontal tissues of smoking cigarettes, cigars, pipes or cannabis are similar. Smokers are 3 times more likely to have a severe form of periodontal disease than non-smokers. Tobacco aggravates periodontal disease by promoting pathogenic bacterial invasion, inhibiting immune defences, aggravating inflammation and increasing alveolar bone loss. Tobacco affects the function and proliferation of periodontal cells, such as periodontal fibroblasts and periodontal ligament cells, and induces apoptosis. Smoking has been shown to interfere with redox homeostasis, alter antioxidant values and negatively influence periodontal disease. [32]

Cementum is synthesised by cementoblasts during the formation of the dental root and plays an essential role in anchoring the tooth to the alveolar bone. Cementoblasts function not only as supporting cells of the periodontium, but also in the maintenance, development and regeneration of periodontal tissues.[32]

Nicotine causes destruction of periodontal tissue directly or through interaction with other factors. One study suggests that nicotine inhibits the migration and proliferation of cementoblasts and induces the synthesis of cytokines and reactive oxygen species by these cells. [32]

Diabetes mellitus:

Type 2 diabetes mellitus is preceded by systemic inflammation leading to decreased pancreatic beta-cell function, apoptosis and insulin resistance. Elevated systemic inflammation leads to entry of periodontal organisms and their virulence factors into the circulation, providing evidence for the effects of periodontitis on diabetes.[32]

The specific mechanism linking diabetes and periodontal disease is not well understood. It is suggested that diabetes is involved in the alteration of the subgingival bacterial community that favours the growth of pathogens. In addition, systemic levels of inflammatory mediators, such as C-reactive protein, TNF-a and IL-6, which are elevated in periodontal disease, could be a link between diabetes and periodontitis. Oxidative stress is likely to be an important link between the two diseases, through the activation of common proinflammatory pathways. [32]

Another mechanism could be interactions between the products of advanced glycosylation and their receptors. Diabetes mellitus is associated with periodontal ligament destruction and tooth loss. [32]

Gingival fluids and saliva have higher concentrations of inflammatory mediators, such as cytokines, among diabetic patients with periodontitis compared to non-diabetics with periodontal disease. [32]

According to the European Federation of Periodontology and the American Academy of Periodontology, a dose-response relationship was identified between the severity of periodontal disease and the adverse consequences of diabetes and that periodontal treatment was beneficial as an anti-diabetic medication. [32]

Stress:

Stress reduces salivary secretions and promotes dental plaque formation. A positive association has been observed between stress scores and salivary stress markers: cortisol, beta and alpha amylase endorphin, tooth loss and probing depth of 5-8 mm. [32]

It was indicated that stress is related to the immune system and different immunological changes occur in response to different stressful events. Chronic stress causes destruction of the periodontium in susceptible individuals. However, the complex biological nature of stress limits the understanding of how it modulates periodontal health, which is further hampered by other environmental factors at work. [32]

Depressed individuals have a higher concentration of cortisol in gingival crevicular fluid and respond less well to periodontal treatment. Academic stress also causes poor oral hygiene and gingival inflammation, with increased IL-1ß concentration.

Genetic factor:

As already mentioned, the presence of bacteria is fundamental for the development of the disease, however, the existence of other factors favour its onset and progression, such as the patient's immune response. There are patients who, despite having acceptable plaque control and not smoking, have more severe disease than patients with worse plaque control and who smoke. This raises the underlying role of genetic susceptibility. Added to this is the fact that periodontal destruction is often observed in members of the same family and in different generations of the same family, suggesting a genetic basis related to susceptibility for periodontal disease.

Other local and systemic factors influencing the development of periodontopathies:

Dental tartar, calculus or tartar, poor oral hygiene, abnormal occlusal forces, food packing, unreplaced missing teeth, stomatological iatrogenies, malocclusions, injurious habits, bruxism, alterations of dental, gingival and bone morphology.[7]

Diagnosis of chronic periodontal disease:

Periodontal diseases do not usually cause severe pain or discomfort. The most common symptom is spontaneous bleeding during tooth brushing, although this is less evident in patients who smoke. Pus may also appear on the gums, bad taste or bad breath, reddening of the gums, receding gums and the appearance of longer teeth, spaces between the teeth or changes in their position, hypersensitivity to thermal changes, especially cold, pain and mobility of the teeth .[27]

The diagnosis of certainty can only be made by the dentist or periodontist using a probe. It assesses whether the periodontal tissues are inflamed on the surface: gingivitis and whether there has been a loss of the supporting tissues: periodontitis. X-rays may also be necessary to confirm the findings. Diagnosis can be complemented by microbiological analysis to identify pathogenic bacteria, or by genetic analysis to assess the individual's susceptibility to the disease. [27]

The diagnosis of periodontal disease is of vital importance as it is the starting point for providing better treatment to patients. To do this, a good clinical history must be taken, using diagnostic tools such as the periodontal probe, clinical and radiographic preservation, in order to determine abnormalities in the tone and consistency of the gum, to observe whether there is gingival displacement, and also to check each of the teeth to detect whether there is any mobility in them. [35,36]

Clinical features of chronic periodontal disease:

Its main clinical manifestations include spontaneous bleeding or reddening of the gums, tooth mobility or tooth separation, gingival recession, ulceration, gingival abscess, periodontal pocket formation, bad breath, hypersensitivity to cold, chewing dysfunction and tooth loss. [20,28]

Furthermore, periodontitis is associated with a negative impact on people's quality of life, producing different effects on patients including: impairment, discomfort, discomfort, limitation of masticatory function; it also affects patients' appearance, self-esteem and psychosocial well-being. [20]

Classification of chronic periodontal disease:

The world's two leading scientific associations in periodontology, the American Academy of Periodontology and the European Federation of Periodontology, have joined forces to develop a new classification system for periodontal diseases and conditions in 2018 that will adapt to current scientific knowledge and attempt to address some of the limitations and application problems of the previous classification system.[37]

As a significant example of this process, the changes in the classification of periodontitis are highly relevant. In the previous, internationally accepted classification of 1999, periodontitis was subdivided into: chronic periodontitis, aggressive periodontitis, periodontitis as a manifestation of systemic disease, necrotising periodontal diseases and periodontal abscesses. Although this classification structure was widely used in both clinical practice and research for almost 20 years, it lacked a clear pathobiologically based distinction between the described categories, which led to difficulties in establishing a clear diagnosis and thus in the specific implementation of preventive and therapeutic measures in these specific clinical entities. Since this 1999 workshop, substantial new information has emerged that has evaluated the differential characteristics of genetic susceptibility, microbial aggression and host response in these clinical entities, but this evidence was not able to differentiate clear phenotypes that would allow a clear distinction between the pathologies and conditions that had been defined. Similarly, they were unable to identify specific disease patterns; nor did the impact of environmental and systemic risk factors significantly alter the expression of periodontitis. A similar discussion was conducted on gingival pathologies and periodontal manifestations of systemic diseases and developmental and acquired disorders. Peri-implant diseases and conditions were also classified. [38, 39, 40, 41,42] Classification of gingival health and plaque-induced gingival disorders: Periodontal health:

Clinical health with a healthy periodontium.

Clinical gingival health with a reduced periodontium.

Patient with stable periodontitis.

Patient without periodontitis.

Plaque-induced gingivitis:

Intact periodontium.

Reduced periodontium in a patient without periodontitis.

Reduced periodontium in successfully treated periodontitis patients.

Exclusively associated with biofilm.

Mediated by systemic or local risk factors.

Systemic risk factors, modifying factors:

Smoking.

Hyperglycaemia.

Nutritional factors.

Pharmacological agents.

Steroid sex hormones.

Puberty.

Menstrual cycle.

Pregnancy.

Oral contraceptives.

Haematological disorders.

Local risk factors, predisposing factors:

Plaque/biofilm retentive factors such as restorations.

Dry mouth.

Drug-induced gingival hypertrophy. [37]

Periodontal disease classification systems group conditions ranging from gingivitis to the various stages of periodontitis and now peri-implant conditions. These have been modified and updated to enable clinicians to make appropriate diagnoses and provide optimal treatment. Since the first description of periodontal disease, different classification systems have been used to group them according to their aetiology, pathogenesis, location and progression, but there is always some particularity or complication to make the appropriate and personalised diagnosis of patients. [43, 44,45]

Classification in force in Cuba:

Chronic:

Superficial:

Oedematous, fibrous and fibroedematous gingivitis.

Chronic desquamative gingivitis. [7]

Deep:

Adult periodontitis.

Pre-pubertal periodontitis.

Localised and generalised juvenile periodontitis.

Rapidly progressive periodontitis.[7]

The most common conditions that occur in these tissues are chronic immuno-inflammatory conditions such as gingivitis and periodontitis, which, when left untreated, lead more or less rapidly to tooth loss. Gingivitis is characterised by reversible gingival inflammation without evidence of periodontal breakdown. Over time, untreated gingivitis can progress to destructive periodontitis. [22,27] Chronic gingivitis:

Gingivitis is inflammation of the gingiva and is characterised by changes in colouring, commonly from pale pink to bright red, oedema and bleeding, as well as altered tissue consistency. These changes are the result of the accumulation of dental plaque along the gingival margin and the inflammatory response of the immune system to the presence of bacterial products. [28]

In this case the junctional epithelium does not migrate, i.e. if there is a pathological increase in the depth of the gingival sulcus called a pocket this is at the expense of the coronary migration of the margin, therefore, when referring to chronic gingivitis with pockets, these are: Virtual, False, Relative or Gingival. Chronic gingivitis is more frequent in children and young people. [7]

Classification of chronic gingivitis:

Chronic gingivitis is classified according to the groups of teeth affected: Localised: When it affects one tooth or group of teeth.

Generalised: When it covers a whole jaw or the whole mouth.[7]

Another way of classifying gingivitis is according to the different areas of the gum that are affected:

Marginal gingivitis

Papillary gingivitis

Diffuse gingivitis

Chronic marginal gingivitis: this is where changes in morphology are observed in the marginal or free gingiva, papillary gingivitis: this is confined to the interdental papilla. When both margin and papilla are affected, it is also called marginal, although some clinicians prefer to call it marginal-papillary. It is considered diffuse: when the inflammatory process involves the gums: marginal or free, papillary and inserted or adherent.[7] According to the clinical characteristics and histopathological image anatomical-clinical aspect, chronic gingivitis can be classified as follows:

Chronic oedematous gingivitis: The gingiva is smooth, shiny, bluish-red in colour and soft in consistency, the interdental sulcus and marginal sulcus are erased. The bevelled shape of the gingiva becomes rounded. If the inflammatory process reaches the attached gingiva, the gingival stippling is lost. Bleeding occurs at the slightest stimulation.[7]

Chronic fibrous gingivitis: The gingiva is firm, normal or slightly lighter in colour and hard in consistency. There is loss of normal bevelling with increased gingival volume. There is no loss of stippling, occasionally there may be reinforcement of the stippling. Bleeding is less marked. [7]

Chronic fibroedematous gingivitis: Clinically we can find clinical changes of oedematous and fibrous gingivitis. The gingiva may be soft and not hypercoloured or red and firm in consistency, bleeding is not abundant. [7]

Chronic desquamative gingivitis: a peculiar lesion of the gingiva characterised by intense reddening and desquamation of the surface epithelium, not a specific entity, but rather a non-specific gingival manifestation of a variety of systemic disorders. [7]

Chronic periodontitis:

Chronic inflammatory periodontal disease periodontitis is the leading cause of tooth loss in adults, thus the absence of dental organs affects the function of the stomatognathic system and can be a risk factor for multiple local and systemic conditions. Periodontitis is a chronic, non-communicable, inflammatory and infectious disease. It is characterised by gingival inflammation that extends beyond the gingiva and causes irreversible breakdown of root-bound connective tissue and resorption of alveolar bone. Progressive destruction of the connective tissue and alveolar bone results in apical migration of the gingival epithelium and pocket formation. Ultimately, the destruction of the periodontium leads to tooth mobility, reduced masticatory function and eventual tooth loss. It is a chronic disease that progresses through crises with similar clinical expression and a shared chain of pathogenic events, but varying in aetiology and prognosis. Tissue destruction in chronic periodontitis usually occurs slowly and progressively, without causing great discomfort, and tooth loss occurs several years after the onset of the disease. The disease produces inflammatory and infectious reactions at the local level, i.e. the periodontium, and at the systemic level, with a high impact on the general health of the patient. Periodontitis can be considered a public health problem because in addition to affecting oral health, in the last decade it has been suggested as a risk indicator. [30, 46, 47,48]

General clinical features of chronic periodontitis: Presence of chronic gingival inflammation.

Gingival bleeding.

Presence of supraosseous or infraosseous real bags.

Periodontal recession.

Purulent exudate.

Tooth mobility.

Pathological migration.

Halitosis.

Loss of attachment and supporting bone. [7]

Different forms of presentation have been described, based mainly on the age of onset and aggressiveness of the disease. [22]

Classification of chronic periodontitis:

Prepubertal periodontitis: This term describes a disease that begins during or after the eruption of the primary teeth at 4 or 5 years of age and less than 12 years of age. The disease affects both sexes equally and usually has a genetic basis. Periodontal lesions can be localised or generalised, and are more common in upper teeth than lower teeth.[7]

Juvenile periodontitis: this is an unusual form of periodontitis, early and severe, which generally appears between 12 and 26 years of age, affecting both sexes, although in some studies a slight predominance of the female sex has been observed. It is characterised by the fact that the gums do not show any ostensible clinical changes in colour or texture; if these are present, they are not alarming, but there are deep periodontal pockets with great connective and osseous destruction. [7] Rapidly progressive periodontitis: a group of periodontitis characterised by rapid and progressive destruction of the clinical attachment and alveolar bone. [7]

Chronic periodontitis: Chronic periodontitis is the least aggressive form, later in adulthood and is the most common form. Cyclical patterns of exacerbations and remissions, i.e. periods of quiescence and periods of disease activity, are suggested and there is no consensus on the cause of this mode of progression, what is clear is that it can take years to progress.[7, 22] Chronic periodontitis is the best known and most common form of periodontitis, almost always starting in young adulthood and progressing throughout the individual's life.

Chronic periodontitis can affect the entire dentition but, in general, molars and incisors are more susceptible, while upper and lower canines and lower first premolars are more resistant to the disease.[7]

Chronic periodontitis is subclassified according to its degree of progression: Mild periodontitis:

When there is gingival inflammation, with periodontal pocket formation, bleeding on probing, horizontal bone loss, less than 1/3 of the root length, and possible grade 1 tooth mobility. [7]

Moderate periodontitis:

The periodontal pocket may be supra-osseous or infra-osseous, bone loss may be up to 1/3 of the root length, there is eventual grade 1 or 2 tooth mobility. Occasionally there may be grade I furcation injury. [7]

Severe, severe or complicated periodontitis:

It has the same characteristics as moderate furcation, only the bone loss is greater than 1/3 of the length of the root, and can be either horizontal or angular. The furcation lesion may be grade I or II, with possible grade 2 or 3 mobility. [7]

Treatment of chronic periodontal disease:

In the treatment of periodontal diseases, such as gingivitis, it is necessary to clean the bacteria that have accumulated by removing dental plaque and dental calculus, also called tartar, which is mineralised plaque. As a preventive measure, teeth and gums should be brushed to keep them clean and healthy. The treatment of periodontitis is organised in two phases. In the first phase, also called the basic phase of treatment, bacteria will be removed from the periodontal pockets by scaling and root planing, which involves cleaning bacteria, plaque and calculus from the roots of the teeth. Sometimes this phase of treatment is accompanied by the use of antibiotics. However, in aggressive or advanced disease, a second phase of treatment is necessary, which consists of accessing these deep periodontal pockets. This phase is called periodontal surgery. Sometimes localised bone regeneration techniques can also be applied during periodontal surgery. When active treatment ends, the disease should be under control. The maintenance phase continues, which is considered the fundamental phase of periodontal treatment and the only way to achieve long-term control of periodontitis. The basic and surgical phases are very effective in controlling bacteria and achieving periodontal health, but these bacteria tend to recolonise the periodontal pocket from other oral reservoirs and if not properly addressed the disease tends to recur after a few months.

It is important to emphasise that periodontal maintenance is not only a professional prophylaxis or cleaning of the mouth, but an individualised medical action adapted to the needs of each patient. The frequency of maintenance is defined for each individual case, but usually ranges from one visit every 3 months to one every 6 months.

Treatment consists mainly of control of the risk factors and, in severe cases, periodontal surgery, the primary objective of which is not healing but excision of the lesions, which will ensure good subsequent maintenance of the periodontium in the face of the aetiological factors.[30]

One of the procedures that can be used in the treatment of periodontal disease is antibiotic therapy, which consists of providing the patient with medicines that fight the infection caused by the bacteria found in the periodontal tissues, which can be very varied. [49]

Antibiotics used in the therapy of periodontal disease: In cases of diagnosed gingivitis, the American Dental Association suggests that in addition to the mechanical methods used for plaque control, other types of agents should be applied to help reduce inflammation, the main ones being chlorhexidine and triclosan. Anti-plaque agents that are used correctly contribute to the treatment to reduce gingival inflammation in patients who do not perform adequate cleaning, however, the effect of the adjuvant substances would only occur on supragingival plaque. [49]

Due to the variety of antibiotics available, it is possible to use a few types, depending on the case at hand. One of the groups used is the tetracyclines, which are effective against Gram-negative bacteria such as Agregatibacter actinomycetencomitans.[49]

Metronidazole is a bactericidal drug that acts selectively on anaerobic bacteria such as Prevotella intermedia, Fusobacterium nucleatum and Bacteroides. [49]

Amoxicillin together with clavulanic acid is used against strict anaerobic bacteria, which are present in advanced periodontal disease. [49]

Clindamycin is a macrolide whose action is bacteriostatic and acts on subunit 50 causing alteration in the protein synthesis of the bacterial cell, its spectrum includes microorganisms such as Prevotella intermedia and Fusobacterium nucleatum. [49]

Prevention of periodontal disease:

Prevention of a common disease such as periodontal disease is very complicated because of its multifactorial nature, involving genetics, environment, social status and other factors. Preventive actions are aimed at stopping the progression of gingival and periodontal diseases or preventing their occurrence in the supposedly healthy or at-risk population. The best way to prevent periodontitis is to maintain proper oral hygiene to control plaque levels; predisposed individuals may develop the disease despite proper oral hygiene. Personal oral hygiene should be accompanied by regular visits to the dentist or periodontist in order to make an early diagnosis of the disease. Lifestyle changes are then necessary. Medications that reduce salivary secretion or cause gingival hypertrophy should be avoided or used with caution, as they facilitate periodontal disease. Patients with chronic stressful situations should be evaluated by qualified personnel for effective anti-stress measures. Adequate control of diabetes mellitus and other systemic diseases reduces the risk of onset and progression of periodontal diseases.[27, 30]

**Osteoarticular diseases:**

The importance of bones in the body is paramount, as they, along with the muscles, are responsible for the movement of the body, as well as providing solid protection for vital organs such as the heart, brain and lungs. Also within the bones is the bone marrow, which is essential for the production of various types of blood cells. Bone cells are continuously regenerating, which means that every decade, all 206 bones in our body are completely renewed. There are multiple diseases that affect the bone system, in its morphology and physiology, which can cause chronic pain and inflammation, weakness, immobility, and fractures, among other symptoms. Dysfunction of the system formed by bones and joints is an anomaly of frequent clinical presentation and also one of the most frequent causes of consultation in Primary Care. [50]

Osteoarticular disorders generally include the following clinical pictures: degenerative rheumatisms such as osteoarthritis, which is the most common osteoarticular disorder, inflammatory joint and soft tissue rheumatisms such as rheumatoid arthritis, inflammatory spondyloarthropathies such as ankylosing spondylitis and other arthritis, metabolic rheumatisms such as osteoporosis, which is becoming increasingly important today, or gout, and extra-articular rheumatisms such as fibromyalgia. Fibromyalgia and rheumatoid arthritis are the most frequent rheumatic problems after osteoarthritis, although with a notable difference. [50]

The increase in life expectancy has increased the elderly population, favouring an increase in the incidence of degenerative bone and joint diseases. Osteoarticular disorders are characterised by pain and functional impotence of some part of the locomotor system. Thus, they are considered one of the most prevalent causes of symptomatology and functional limitation. In the active population, they are one of the most important causes of work absenteeism and permanent disability with a growing economic repercussion, generating great demand for care and the consumption of medicines. It interferes with the functional capacity and quality of life of patients. An action for them is to prevent their progression as they lead to chronicity and disability. Osteoarthritis is considered the second most disabling condition after cardiovascular diseases. [51]

The most prevalent osteoarticular diseases are:

Rheumatoid arthritis and osteoporosis.

**Rheumatoid arthritis:**

Rheumatoid arthritis is a chronic, autoimmune rheumatic disease that causes joint inflammation, pain, deformity and difficulty in movement. It predominantly affects women. It can have extra-articular behaviour and damage organs and systems such as the heart, kidney and lung. For this reason, it is considered to be a systemic disease.[52]

It affects some joints more severely than others, mainly the more mobile joints, such as the hands and feet, elbows, shoulders, hips, knees and ankles. On the other hand, there are others that are never affected. If the inflammation remains over time and is not controlled, it can end up damaging the bones, ligaments and tendons around the joint. This can lead to progressive joint deformity and loss of capacity. This has a very negative impact on patients' quality of life.[52]

Causes of rheumatoid arthritis:

The cause of the onset of this disease is unknown. It is known to be an autoimmune process. The genetic component is also very relevant. There are also external factors; the first and most frequent is smoking, but there may be others, such as certain infections, periodontitis and obesity. The intestinal microbiota and diet can also influence its appearance. [52]

Symptoms of rheumatoid arthritis:

The disease often begins slowly and insidiously with general manifestations of other diseases, such as fever or asthenia. The main symptom of the disease is joint involvement, which is evident through pain and swelling. Other manifestations may also appear, such as joint stiffness or numbness after prolonged rest, especially when getting up in the morning, which gradually disappears as the patient carries out daily activities, as well as muscle weakness and limited mobility. If the disease is in an advanced stage, the patient may have some deformity due to the progressive deterioration of the affected joints. In addition, it may progress and affect vital organs such as the kidney or lung. [52]

It often causes dryness of the skin and mucous membranes. This results in inflammation and subsequent atrophy of the glands that produce tears, saliva, digestive juices or vaginal discharge known as Sjögren's syndrome. It can also cause some fever and sometimes inflammation of the blood vessels: vasculitis, leading to nerve damage or sores on the legs called ulcers. [52]

Other symptoms include inflammation of the membranes lining the lungs, pleuritis or the lining of the heart, pericarditis, or inflammation and scarring of the lungs can lead to chest pain, shortness of breath and abnormal heart function. [52]

Diagnosis of rheumatoid arthritis:

There are no specific tests to diagnose rheumatoid arthritis, but rheumatologists can determine its existence through a combination of a clinical interview in which the patient is asked about symptoms, physical examination, patient history and certain tests. Tests such as :

Blood tests. [5]

Rheumatoid factor tests: Test for antibodies to citrullinated peptides. These antibodies are present in two thirds of patients with this pathology. [52]

X-rays to detect the presence of joint erosions.

Treatments for rheumatoid arthritis:

Rheumatoid arthritis is a chronic disease for which there is currently no treatment that can cure the condition. [52]

Symptomatic treatments: these are drugs that control only the symptoms. These are painkillers and non-steroidal anti-inflammatory drugs.[52]

Disease-modifying drugs: Disease-modifying drugs have a more profound effect on the mechanisms of pathology. They can be divided into:

Traditional: The most commonly used are methotrexate, leflunomide and sulfasalazine. This group also includes chloroquine and hydroxychloroquine, cyclosporine, azathioprine and minocycline.

Biologics: The most important biologics include: adalimumab, etanercept, columumab, infliximab, abatacept, rituzimab and tocilizumab. [52]

**Osteoporosis:**

Osteoporosis is a systemic skeletal disease characterised by a decrease in bone mass and a deterioration of the microarchitecture of the bones, which leads to an increase in bone fragility and the risk of suffering fractures. This pathology is asymptomatic and can go unnoticed for many years until it finally manifests itself in the form of a fracture. [16]

Causes of osteoporosis:

The origin of osteoporosis must be sought in the factors that influence bone development and bone quality. The risk of osteoporosis will be determined by the maximum level of bone mass attained in adulthood and the decline in bone mass caused by the

26 old age. In addition to ageing, genetic and hereditary factors are involved in its onset. Malnutrition, poor diet, lack of physical exercise and the administration of certain drugs can also favour the appearance of osteoporosis. However, the menopause is one of the most influential factors in the development of osteoporosis in women, as the disappearance of ovarian function causes an increase in bone resorption. The exact role of smoking in osteoporosis is unclear, but a direct link between smoking and decreased bone density has been described. [16] Symptoms of osteoporosis:

For years, osteoporosis has been known as the silent epidemic because this pathology does not produce symptoms, although pain is one of them, which can be diffuse skeletal pain and bone hyperaesthesia, muscle weakness, bone fractures due to microtrauma, with a reduction in the patient's height if there is vertebral crushing. [16]

Types of osteoporosis:

Postmenopausal osteoporosis: the main cause is a lack of oestrogen. Symptoms generally appear in women aged 51 to 75 years, although they may start before or after these ages.[16]

Senile osteoporosis: the result of age-related calcium deficiency and an imbalance between the rate of bone degradation and regeneration. It generally affects people over 70 years of age and is twice as common in women as in men. [16]

Secondary osteoporosis: this can result from certain diseases, such as chronic renal failure and certain hormonal disorders; or from the administration of certain drugs, such as corticosteroids, barbiturates, anticonvulsants and excessive amounts of thyroid hormone. [16]

Diagnosis of osteoporosis:

Based on current knowledge, the diagnostic approach must be carried out on an individual basis, assessing age and other risk factors. In addition, risk factors such as tobacco and alcohol consumption, low weight, family history of osteoporotic fractures, among others, make it possible to identify people at risk of developing the pathology. Therefore, the fundamental basis for diagnosis is based on clinical suspicion.[16]

Treatments for osteoporosis:

The drugs currently used to combat osteoporosis stop bone resorption and prevent bone mineral loss. These are called bone resorption inhibitors and include oestrogens, calcitonins, bisphosphonates such as etidronate, alendronate and risedronate, selective oestrogen receptor modulators such as raloxifene and even statins, drugs that were initially used to combat cholesterol. [16]

Although pharmacological treatment is very important, there are other measures aimed at correcting nutritional deficiencies and improving lifestyle that can prevent falls and minimise the intensity of the impact of the disease, the most important being that the patient takes the necessary amounts of calcium and vitamin D. [16]

Lifestyle modification: experts recommend avoiding immobility and following physiotherapeutic guidelines that limit deformity and pain, as well as abstaining from smoking and drinking large amounts of alcohol. [16]

Physical exercise: sport increases bone mass during growth in children and adolescents and can also help to reduce bone loss in older people. [16]

**Relationship between chronic periodontal disease and osteoarticular diseases:**

Therefore, taking into account the high frequency of oral and rheumatic diseases in the population worldwide, the possible pathogenic interrelationship between the two diseases due to shared inflammatory precursors. [53]

Oral microbiota can cause oral inflammation, but can also directly contribute to systemic inflammation, which may increase the risk of developing or worsening systemic diseases. Different periodontal periodontopathogens have been associated with the pathogenesis of different diseases by being found in disease-specific lesions, such as atherosclerosis, Alzheimer's disease or rheumatoid arthritis. [54, 55,56]

Relationship between chronic periodontal disease and rheumatoid arthritis:

Chronic periodontal disease and rheumatoid arthritis are two chronic systemic inflammatory diseases of multifactorial origin commonly diagnosed in the elderly. Both diseases are characterised by chronic inflammation, bone destruction, soft tissue damage, similar cellular and humoral immune response and a common genetic background. The relationship between periodontitis and rheumatoid arthritis is given by the significant and constant increase of genetic and inflammatory mediators as well as microbial products: endotoxins. Evaluation of disease activity is essential to make therapeutic decisions and to establish the prognosis of patients with rheumatoid arthritis.[52, 53, 57,58, 59, 60,61]

Periodontal disease and rheumatoid arthritis are two inflammatory diseases with a common pathogenesis. This link between the two diseases is thought to be bidirectional, i.e. patients with rheumatoid arthritis would have a higher incidence of periodontal disease and vice versa. [53]

Both rheumatoid arthritis and periodontal disease have many common pathological features shown below:

Inflammatory relationship between the two diseases:

Chronic inflammation, such as that seen in periodontal disease, produces a systemic inflammatory burden that can affect other systemic conditions. In fact, many authors conclude that inflammation must be the link between periodontal disease and rheumatoid arthritis. [53]

The inflammatory mechanisms of periodontal disease result in periodontal soft tissue and bone destruction similar to the pattern of joint destruction in rheumatoid arthritis. In addition, both processes show an exaggerated inflammatory reaction, regulated by the infiltration of immune cells, enzymes and cytokines. So much so, that it has been proposed that the relationship is produced by a mechanism that has been called the double knock model, in which a first knock would be an extrasynovial inflammation as may occur in periodontal disease, followed by a second knock in which an exacerbated response would be induced in the joints producing rheumatoid arthritis. Likewise, smoking has also been proposed as a possible factor producing the first stroke. Tobacco, which is a risk factor in both rheumatoid arthritis and periodontal disease, has the ability to produce citrullinated proteins, which in susceptible individuals, could result in the production of anti-citrullinated protein antibodies that years later, in a second hit, would lead to arthritis by provoking an immune response in the synovial membrane of the joints. It is suspected that there may be individuals who have an inflammatory phenotype, with a predisposition to various inflammatory conditions. [53]

In these two pathologies, there is an exaggerated inflammatory reaction that results in activation of the complement system and the production of proinflammatory mediators, cytokines and substances that lead to the destruction of soft tissue and bone around the teeth and joints, as well as their chronification. It has also been suggested that periodontal microvascular alterations may play a role in the relationship between the two diseases, as rheumatoid arthritis patients have a characteristic periodontal blood microcirculation. Abnormalities found in rheumatoid arthritis patients consisted of small elongated loops, microhaemorrhages, low-density capillaries and visible subcapillary alterations in the venous plexus. Hypotheses on the pathogenic mechanism of vascular damage propose that the precipitation of circulating autoantibodies and immune complexes in vessel walls, considered the main causes of damage, occurs. Vascular damage correlates with the production of osteopretogerin by endothelial cells, although this is necessary for good vascular homeostasis. [53]

Role of periodontopathogenic bacteria:

Local infection leading to inflammation in periodontal disease has been proposed as a possible trigger mechanism for systemic inflammatory processes or spread of infection. Porphyromonas gingivalis, Tannarella forsythia and Treponema denticola play an important role in activating periodontal destruction; they initiate an immune response mediated by neutrophils, monocytes and T and B lymphocytes. [62, 63, 64]

During inflammation, peptide or protein citrullination takes place, which is the conversion of the amino acid arginine to citrulline and occurs under the action of the enzyme peptidyl arginine deaminase. This enzyme induces citrullination of certain proteins into antigens, which are recognised by anti-cyclic citrullinated peptide antibodies. These antibodies are specific markers of rheumatoid arthritis and are found in 80% of patients with a specificity of 99%. They are produced in the inflamed synovial membrane. Studies show that levels of these antibodies are significantly higher in rheumatoid arthritis patients with advanced periodontal disease than in rheumatoid arthritis patients without periodontal disease.[64, 65, 66,67]

Peptidyl arginine deaminase is an enzyme expressed by inflammatory cells: T and B lymphocytes, neutrophils, eosinophils, monocytes, NK cells and synovial membrane macrophages, and also by the bacterium Porphyromonas gingivalis. In turn, Porphyromonas gingivalis is the only bacterium that expresses the enzyme peptidyl arginine deaminase. This is indicative of the concept that infection with this organism may induce or accelerate rheumatoid arthritis by facilitating antigen and antibody production. Antibodies against Porphyromonas gingivalis are found in higher concentrations in patients with rheumatoid arthritis, and this is related to the presence of anti-cyclic citrullinated peptide antibodies. The presence of antibodies to this bacterium in serum and synovial fluid and their identification in DNA in rheumatoid arthritis patients reinforces this hypothesis.[67] In addition, the proinflammatory cytokines IL-23 and IL-17 and their receptors also play an important role in the immunopathology of these diseases. IL-23 activates and expands Th17 clones through IL-23R and promotes the production of IL-17 and RANKL; however, soluble IL-23R can block the IL-23 receptor by inhibiting IL-23 signalling. IL-17 through IL-17RA can activate fibroblasts and macrophages expressing RANKL which activates osteoclast precursors and initiates bone erosion in joints and alveolar bone. Like the soluble IL-23R receptor, soluble IL-17RA can block IL-17A and inhibit its signalling.[67] Other biochemical markers:

c-reactive protein is an acute phase protein that is synthesised in the liver and is elevated in serum under inflammatory conditions. It has been used as a marker of inflammation associated with rheumatoid arthritis and it has been proposed that it may be increased in patients with periodontal disease, although there is a low level of evidence for this claim. [68]

Rheumatoid factor is a non-specific antibody used in the diagnosis of rheumatoid arthritis, although there are 15% of patients with rheumatoid arthritis who do not manifest this marker. The presence of this marker has been studied in patients with periodontal disease, although no statistically significant evidence has been demonstrated in patients with rheumatoid arthritis and periodontal disease. The erythrocyte sedimentation rate is a technique used to determine the presence of systemic inflammation and has been used as a diagnostic aid in determining rheumatoid arthritis.[68]

Common pathways of tissue destruction:

Chronic periodontal disease shows a common inflammatory profile with rheumatoid arthritis, presenting similar patterns of hard and soft tissue destruction. Similarities between them appear at the molecular and cellular level. [68]

Persistently elevated levels of proinflammatory cytokines such as IL-1 beta, IL-6 and

TNF-alpha and low levels of anti-inflammatory cytokines such as IL-10 correlate with hard and soft tissue destruction in joints and alveolar bone in rheumatoid arthritis and periodontal disease respectively. We know that there is increased expression of IL-1, 6, 8 and TNF-alpha where Porphyromonas gingivalis is present. [68]

IL-17 has been particularly prominent in the pathogenesis of rheumatoid arthritis. It is produced by T-helper 17 cells and induces the release of inflammatory mediators including those responsible for the destruction of bone and synovial cartilage. TH 17 and IL-17 cells have been identified in chronic periodontal disease, and the bacterium Porphyromonas gingivalis stimulates their expression. [68]

Common genetic factors:

It has been suggested that both diseases share a genetic link and some authors suggest that antibodies developed during periodontal infection or the periodontal pathogen itself lead to the development of rheumatoid arthritis.[68]

The most important correlation between periodontal disease and rheumatoid arthritis is associated with the HLA-DRB1 gene. The shared epitope is a group of alleles of the major histocompatibility complex and is the strongest genetic risk factor for rheumatoid arthritis, and appears in the same alleles that have been linked to rapid progression of periodontal disease, indicating that the two diseases may share common immunogenetic features. [68]

Common risk factors:

The most common risk factors influencing both diseases are:

- Tobacco.
- Age and immunodeficiency: Age deteriorates the immune system leading to a compromise that causes progressive deterioration in both periodontal disease and rheumatoid arthritis.
- Exposure to microorganisms: Increased levels of Porphyromonas gingivalis have been seen in adults over 60 years of age with chronic periodontal disease.
- Stress and low socioeconomic status: stress causes dysregulation of the immune system through complex interactions with the neuroendocrine axis. In periodontal disease, this factor, in addition to generating a direct alteration of the immune response, can intervene through unhealthy behaviours, which increase the risk of developing periodontal disease. In many patients, it has been observed that the first manifestations and symptomatic flare-ups of rheumatoid arthritis are preceded by periods of stress or increased smoking. [68]

Common therapy in both diseases:

There are several therapies used in the treatment of rheumatoid arthritis that have a beneficial effect on periodontal disease:

· Nonsteroidal anti-inflammatory drugs: Systemic nonsteroidal anti-inflammatory drugs, such as naproxen, when administered daily for three years significantly reduce alveolar bone loss and pain and inflammation in rheumatoid arthritis.

· Corticosteroids: Inhibit inflammatory cytokines such as IL-1, 8 and TNF-alpha, reducing the inflammatory response in both diseases.

· Antirheumatic drugs: They mitigate the symptoms of rheumatoid arthritis and may affect the progression of bone loss, but do not improve periodontal symptoms. A drawback of their use is toxicity, so they have been restricted for the treatment of periodontal disease.

· Anti-TNF-alpha agents: Used in the treatment of rheumatoid arthritis, they show therapeutic efficacy in this disease, and also show beneficial effects in periodontal disease.

· Other anticytokine agents are beneficial in rheumatoid arthritis, but have not been tested in periodontal disease.

· Tetracyclines: Doxycycline in subantimicrobial doses has been approved for the modulation of periodontal disease. In rheumatoid arthritis, it produces good results in combination with methotrexate. Low-dose doxycycline is safe and effective in periodontal disease. At low doses with methotrexate it improves the severity of rheumatoid arthritis.

· Bisphosphonates: Prevent bone destruction in both diseases. [68]

Non-surgical periodontal therapy:

Treatment of periodontal disease by reducing or eliminating the source of infection can play a key role in reducing the risk and severity of rheumatoid arthritis. In rheumatoid arthritis, physical disability at the level of the phalanges hinders oral hygiene and promotes periodontal disease. [68]

Non-surgical periodontal treatment in rheumatoid arthritis patients with moderate to severe chronic periodontal disease reduces the severity of rheumatoid arthritis by reducing systemic inflammatory mediators, especially TNF-alpha. Scaling and root planing reduces exposure to bacteria and their toxins, thus improving rheumatoid arthritis. Therefore, non-surgical periodontal treatment of patients with moderate-severe periodontal disease reduces the severity of rheumatoid arthritis. [68]

Clinical evidence of the relationship between the diseases:

A relationship between rheumatoid arthritis and periodontal disease has been found based on altered clinical periodontal indices in patients with rheumatoid arthritis. It is thought that patients with rheumatoid arthritis may have a significantly higher incidence of alveolar bone loss; they also appear to have more missing teeth than non-diseased patients with the same degree of periodontal disease, which may be due to less conservative treatment in patients with rheumatoid arthritis due to their delicate health status. Similarly, it has been suggested that these patients may have greater difficulty in maintaining adequate oral hygiene, however, this lack of oral hygiene could only partially explain the relationship between these two diseases. Among the clinical parameters studied, the first is the bacterial plaque index, where there is great variability in the results. An increase in the amount of bacterial plaque has been found in patients with rheumatoid arthritis compared to patients without the disease. [69]

Tooth loss has also been studied and found to be higher in patients with rheumatoid arthritis. The relationship between the severity of periodontitis and rheumatoid arthritis has also been studied. Patients with rheumatoid arthritis have a higher prevalence of periodontal disease, and it has also been shown that these patients are more likely to have a severe form of periodontitis, but the severity and duration of rheumatoid arthritis is independent of the degree of alveolar bone destruction. It is proposed that periodontal disease may worsen the condition of patients with rheumatoid arthritis, justified by the fact that both rheumatoid factor and erythrocyte sedimentation rate decrease when periodontal disease is brought under control. [70]

Relationship between chronic periodontal disease and osteoporosis:

It has been hypothesised that osteoporosis may be a risk factor for periodontal disease and vice versa. There are similarities between the two diseases. Both osteoporosis and periodontal diseases are processes that share pathogenic mechanisms and are determined by a decrease in bone mass and gradual bone resorption; their prevalence increases as the population ages. Their progression or severity can lead to local or systemic involvement. [71]

There are hypothetical models that relate the two conditions: in particular, it is postulated that the reduction in bone mass density related to osteoporosis accelerates alveolar resorption caused by periodontitis by favouring periodontal invasion by bacteria. Invading bacteria would alter the normal homeostasis of bone tissue by increasing the activity of osteoclasts that would reduce bone density locally and systemically, either by direct mechanisms by releasing toxins or indirectly by releasing inflammatory mediators. [71]

The relationship between these two diseases is presented in the following sections: Relationship based on the loss of bone tissue:

The association between these diseases, defined by the loss of bone mass, and alveolar bone loss is evident, although this association is not so clear when osteoporosis is studied in relation to clinical loss of epithelial attachment or probing depth, parameters that mark the existence and severity of periodontal disease. In addition, most of the subjects present with osteoporosis and ostopenia, which makes it difficult to determine the real association between each of these two situations and clinical attachment loss separately, an important fact since, if ostopenia occurs before osteoporosis, we can initiate more active periodontal preventive therapy in patients diagnosed with osteopenia and not wait until they have osteoporosis and probable alveolar bone loss. [71] Relationship based on biomarkers and biofluids;

As mentioned above, osteoporosis affects the jaw bone with a decrease in cortical bone and loss of cancellous bone as well as certain changes in bone microarchitecture that could be implicated in oral health. [71]

The molecular mechanisms underlying this bone loss are related to the decrease in oestrogen that occurs in postmenopausal osteoporosis, are related to the activating receptor ligand for nuclear factor K and B, and the overproduction of certain cytokines with a resorptive effect, such as tumour necrosis factor, and the interleukins IL_1B and IL_6, recently linked to periodontitis. The latter has been considered the most common biomarker in crevicular fluid, giving accurate results and recommending its use as an indicator of periodontal disease progression. The use of paper strips has been found to be the most appropriate and adjusted method for the collection of crevicular fluid, while the enzyme-linked immunosorbent assay can be considered the most conventional method of biofluidic study. [71]

Some of the blood biomarkers used to determine the state of bone remodelling activity and bone loss have also been investigated in body fluids such as saliva and gingival crevicular fluid. However, there are no conclusive studies in this regard, although there is some evidence of an association between osteocalcin at the salivary level and clinical attachment loss. [71]

Relationship of osteoporosis and clinical parameters of periodontitis:

A relationship has been shown between low bone mass and decreased clinical attachment loss, with the highest levels of clinical attachment loss occurring in those with lower bone density and increased gingival recession. [71]

In women of menopausal age where osteoporosis is a predominant disease, a direct relationship between severe clinical attachment loss and low bone density was observed. They also had significantly higher pocket depth and interproximal alveolar bone loss compared to the non-osteoporotic group. [71]

Also the presence or absence of subgingival plaque is associated with bone mineral density and the amelocemental boundary. [72]

Osteoporosis is often present in patients with poor oral hygiene and severe periodontitis, concluding that osteoporosis is an important risk factor for periodontal disease and appears to act as a driver of periodontal disease.[73,74]

Treatments used to prevent osteoporosis have also been shown to have a positive effect on periodontal health. The use of vitamin D, calcium supplements and hormone therapy are shown to be beneficial in increasing mandibular bone mass. [74]

## Methodological design:

A descriptive observational cross-sectional study was carried out. In the Stomatological Service of the Nguyen Van Troi Polyclinic from January 2023 to May 2024. The population ranged in age from 51 to 70 years and gave informed consent (Appendix 1) to participate in the study. The sample was obtained by simple random sampling and consisted of 32 patients.

## Inclusion criteria:

Patients presenting with a medical diagnosis of rheumatoid arthritis or osteoporosis and who were diagnosed with gingivitis and/or periodontitis on clinical stomatological examination.

## Exclusion criteria:

Patients with another medical diagnosis that differs from rheumatoid arthritis or osteoporosis.

## Methodology and methods:

Methods:

Empirical*:* Based on daily practice, experience and observation of the facts, it allowed the final report to be drawn up. The form was aimed at determining the exact symptoms and characteristics of the pathologies in each patient. (Annex 2) Statistical*:* This method was used for data processing.

Methodology:

Based on a medical diagnosis of an osteoarticular disease, a form was created according to the clinical stomatological diagnosis, which made it possible to describe the relationship between the chronic periodontal diseases and the osteoarticular diseases referred to.

For the diagnosis of periodontal diseases in terms of gingivitis and periodontitis, a thorough clinical examination was carried out, supported by the use of a periodontal probe to check for bleeding, presence or absence of pockets; tooth mobility was checked with the use of X-rays that made it possible to appreciate **the** presence or absence of bone damage.

## Operationalisation of the variables:

Age: according to age at the time of the study.

- 51 - 55 years.
- 56 - 60 years.
- 61 - 65 years.
- 66 - 70 years.

Sex: according to biological gender.

- Male.
- Female.

Clinical signs of chronic periodontal disease: according to clinical features of periodontal diseases in relation to osteoarticular diseases.

- Gingivorrhoea
- Real bags
- Virtual stock exchanges
- Bone loss
- Tooth mobility

Bone loss: the X-ray determines the existence of bone loss and establishes its quantity, distribution and type. It can be of type:

- Horizontal: perpendicular to the major axis of the tooth.
- Vertical, angular or oblique: angular or oblique to the tooth axis.

Tooth mobility: according to Laura Lau's criteria:

- Grade 0: corresponds to a tooth with no mobility.
- Grade 1: corresponds to minimal mobility, approximately 1 mm in the lingual vestibule or palatal direction.
- Grade 2: mobility is more than 1 mm in the vestibulo-lingual or palatal direction.
- Grade 3: is mobility of 2 mm or more in the vestibulo-lingual or palatal direction, coupled with intrusive movement.
- Grade 4: the tooth has no anchorage at all in the socket, it is retained only by the gingiva.

Actual pockets: pathological deepening of the gingival sulcus due to destruction of the supporting tissues of the tooth and migration of the junctional epithelium in the apical direction. The depth of the pockets at probing was taken into account:

- 3 mm
- 4 to 5 mm
- Bowl > 6 mm

Risk factors: common to both diseases.

- PDB: presence of Dentobacterial Plaque
- Smoking: patients who are regular smokers
- Stress: patients who report being under stressful situations.
- Immunodeficiency: the presence of immunodeficient diseases causing progressive deterioration in both periodontal disease and bone disease.
- Genetic factor: according to family history of periodontal disease.
- Xerostomia: presence or absence of decreased salivary flow
- Harmful habits: presence or absence of those habits that are capable of influencing both the appearance and evolution as well as the treatment of diseases. Such is the case of unilateral chewing.
- Poor oral hygiene: according to frequency of toothbrushing: 1, 2, 3, 4, 4 or no brushing per day.

Chronic Periodontal Disease: Chronic inflammatory periodontal disease was considered for the study.

- Gingivitis: this is inflammation of the gums and is characterised by changes in colouring, oedema and bleeding, as well as changes in tissue consistency.
- Periodontitis: is a chronic, non-communicable, inflammatory and infectious disease. It is characterised by gingival inflammation that extends beyond the gingiva and causes irreversible rupture of the connective tissue attached to the root and resorption of the alveolar bone.

Osteoarticular diseases: Due to their higher frequency of occurrence in the population, two classifications were used and it was taken into account that the patients only presented one of these two pathologies.

- Osteoporosis: is a systemic skeletal disease characterised by a decrease in bone mass and deterioration of bone microarchitecture.
- Rheumatoid arthritis is a chronic, autoimmune rheumatic disease that causes joint inflammation, pain, deformity and difficulty in movement.

## Data collection techniques:

- Observation: as a technique, it made it possible to obtain data directly from the patient and the pathology that afflicts him or her.
- Direct questioning: this was carried out by means of patient interviews.
- Form (Annex 2): in this case it was fundamental as it provided particular data on each patient that allowed an accurate diagnosis to be made and a relationship to be established between the presence of osteoarticular diseases and periodontal disease.

## Processing methods, data analysis and techniques to be used:

The data were stored in a data file with the professional statistical programme SPSS version 22 on Windows, the information was presented in statistical tables and graphs, in their description absolute frequencies, percentages were calculated. Non-parametric tests such as Chi-square tests for independence of factors were used for the analysis.

## Ethical considerations:

The study was conducted according to international ethical standards for experimental and biomedical human research such as the Nuremberg Code, Declaration of Helsinki I and II, United Nations Principles of Medical Ethics, CIOMS Ethical Guidelines, Universal Declaration on the Human Genome and Human Rights and national ethical standards such as the principles of Medical Ethics. Ethical standards of good practice in human experimentation. These ethical standards were taken into account from the design of the research project and strict compliance was ensured throughout the study process, culminating in the presentation of the results.

The information obtained was used only for this purpose, it was explained to each patient what the study would consist of, it was made clear that it would not involve any harm to their health, in this regard we prepared a model of informed consent (Annex 1), which each patient signed within the basic principles to be taken into account, in order to satisfy the moral, ethical and legal requirements in research with human beings and not to violate the bioethical principles of beneficence, non-maleficence, autonomy and justice.

## Results:

**Table 1.** Distribution according to age and sex in patients with Chronic Periodontal Disease and Osteoarticular Diseases. Nguyen Van Troi Polyclinic. Cascajal. Santo Domingo (January 2023 to May 2024).

| Age | Sex | | | | Total | |
|---|---|---|---|---|---|---|
| | Female | | Male | | | |
| | No. | % | No. | % | No. | % |
| 51 - 55 | 3 | 9,4 | 3 | 9,4 | 6 | 18,8 |
| 56-60 | 4 | 12,5 | 5 | 15,6 | 9 | 28,1 |
| 61-65 | 6 | 18,8 | 4 | 12,5 | 10 | 31,3 |
| 66-70 | 5 | 15,6 | 2 | 6,3 | 7 | 21,9 |
| Total | 18 | 56,3 | 14 | 43,8 | 32 | 100 |

Source: Form

$X^2 = 1.750$ $p = 0.710$ Not significant

A predominance of the female sex was observed with 18 patients, for 56.3% of the total. The male sex was represented by 14 patients for 43.8% of the total. The age groups with the highest representation were 61-65 and 56-60 years with 10 patients in the first group for 31.3% of the total and 9 in the second group for 28.1%. The least represented age group was 51-55 years with 3 female and 3 male patients. The difference between sexes and age groups was not significant.

**Table 2.** Relationship between chronic periodontal disease and gender.

| Disease Chronic Periodontal | Sex | | | | Total | |
|---|---|---|---|---|---|---|
| | Female | | Male | | | |
| | No. | % | No. | % | No. | % |
| Chronic gingivitis | 5 | 15,6 | 6 | 18,8 | 11 | 34,4 |
| Chronic periodontitis | 13 | 40,6 | 8 | 25,0 | 21 | 65,6 |
| Total | 18 | 56,3 | 14 | 43,8 | 32 | 100 |

Source: Form

$X^2 = 0.794$p = 0.465 Not significant

A predominance of chronic periodontitis was observed with 21 patients, for 65.6% of the total, with a higher representation of the female sex with 13 patients, which represented 40.6% of the total. Chronic gingivitis was present in 11 patients, representing 34.4%, and was mostly represented by the male sex with 6 patients for 18.8% of the total. These results showed that patients were more likely to suffer from chronic periodontitis. There was no statistical significance in this case.

**Table 3.** Relationship between chronic periodontal disease and age.

| Age | Chronic Periodontal Disease | | | | Total | |
|---|---|---|---|---|---|---|
| | Chronic gingivitis | | Chronic periodontitis | | | |
| | No. | % | No. | % | No. | % |
| 51 - 55 | 4 | 12,5 | 2 | 6,3 | 6 | 18,8 |
| 56-60 | 3 | 9,4 | 6 | 18,8 | 9 | 28,1 |
| 61-65 | 3 | 9,4 | 7 | 21,9 | 10 | 31,3 |
| 66-70 | 1 | 3,1 | 6 | 18,8 | 7 | 21,9 |
| Total | 11 | 34,4 | 21 | 65,6 | 32 | 100,0 |

Source: Form

$X^2 = 3{,}679$ $p = 0{,}298$ Not significant

The most affected age group with chronic periodontitis was 61-65 years with 7 patients representing 21.9%, followed by 56 - 60 and 66 - 70 years with 6 patients each representing 18.8%. The least representative group in this case was 51-55 years with 2 patients for 6.3%. Chronic gingivitis was mostly represented in the 51-55 years age group with 4 patients representing 12.5%, and was least represented in the 66-70 years age group with only one patient. These results showed that there was a higher frequency of periodontal disease in the 61-65 age group. These data were not statistically significant.

**Table 4.** Relationship between Osteoarticular Diseases and Sex.

| Diseases Osteoarticular | Sex | | | | Total | |
|---|---|---|---|---|---|---|
| | Female | | Male | | | |
| | No. | % | No. | % | No. | % |
| Osteoporosis | 11 | 34,4 | 9 | 28,1 | 20 | 62,5 |
| Rheumatoid arthritis | 7 | 21,9 | 5 | 15,6 | 12 | 37,5 |
| Total | 18 | 56,3 | 14 | 43,8 | 32 | 100 |

Source: Form

X2 = 0,794 p = 0,465 Not significant

A predominance of osteoporosis was observed with 20 patients, for 62.5% of the total, and there was a greater representation in the female sex with 11 patients, which represented 34.4% of the total. Rheumatoid arthritis was present in 12 patients, for 37.5%, and the highest representation was in the female sex with 7 patients for 21.9% of the total. These results showed that the female sex was more prone to suffer from these pathologies due to the hormonal changes that occur in this gender over the years. The values obtained were not significant.

**Table 5.** Relationship between Osteoarticular Diseases and Age.

| Age | Osteoarticular diseases | | | | Total | |
|---|---|---|---|---|---|---|
| | Osteoporosis | | Rheumatoid arthritis | | | |
| | No. | % | No. | % | No. | % |
| 51 - 55 | 4 | 12,5 | 2 | 6,3 | 6 | 18,8 |
| 56-60 | 6 | 18,8 | 3 | 9,4 | 9 | 28,1 |
| 61-65 | 7 | 21,9 | 3 | 9,4 | 10 | 31,3 |
| 66-70 | 3 | 9,4 | 4 | 12,5 | 7 | 21,9 |
| Total | 20 | 62,5 | 12 | 37,5 | 32 | 100 |

Source: Form

$X^2$ = 3,679 p = 0,298 Not significant

The most affected age group with osteoporosis was 61-65 years with 7 patients representing 21.9%, followed by 56 - 60 and 51 - 55 years with 6 and 4 patients respectively representing 18.8% and 12.5%. The least representative group in this case was 66 - 70 years with 3 patients. Rheumatoid arthritis was most represented in the 66-70 age group with 4 patients for 12.5%, and was least represented in the 51-55 age group with 2 patients. The data show that in the age group 61-65 years there was a higher frequency of cases with periodontal disease. The data were not statistically significant.

**Table 6.** Relationship of clinical signs of chronic periodontal disease and osteoarticular diseases.

| Signs of Disease Periodontal Chronicle | Rheumatoid arthritis | | Osteoporosis | | Total | |
|---|---|---|---|---|---|---|
| | No. | % | No. | % | No. | % |
| Gingivorrhoea | 11 | 34,4 | 18 | 56,3 | 29 | 90,6 |
| Virtual Exchanges | 8 | 25 | 3 | 9,4 | 11 | 34,4 |
| Real Bags | 4 | 12,5 | 17 | 53,1 | 21 | 65,6 |
| Bone loss | 4 | 12,5 | 17 | 53,1 | 21 | 65,6 |
| Mobility Dentaria | 4 | 12,5 | 17 | 53,1 | 21 | 65,6 |

Source: Form

X2 = 3.679 p = 0.298 Not significant

The predominant clinical sign was gingivorrhaphy with 29 patients for 90.6 %. In addition, the presence of real pockets, bone loss and tooth mobility were of equal value with 21 patients for 65.6 %, and to a greater extent in the case of osteoporosis with 18 patients for 56.3 %. To a lesser extent was the presence of virtual pockets with 11 patients (34.4%). Thus demonstrating that the fundamental clinical signs of chronic periodontal disease were present in patients with underlying osteoarticular disease. These data were not significant.

**Table 7.** Relationship between bone loss and osteoarticular diseases.

| Bone loss | Rheumatoid arthritis | | Osteoporosis | | Total | |
|---|---|---|---|---|---|---|
| | No | % | No | % | No | % |
| Horizontal | 1 | 4,8 | 2 | 9,5 | 3 | 14,3 |
| Vertical | 3 | 14,3 | 15 | 71,4 | 18 | 85,7 |
| Total | 4 | 19,1 | 17 | 80,9 | 21 | 100 |

Source: Form

$X^2 = 8.875$ $p = 0.003$ Highly Significant

In the analysis of bone loss, bone loss was present in 21 patients. The predominant type of bone loss was vertical or angular with 18 patients (85.7%) and horizontal bone loss in only 3 patients (14.3%). The presence of bone loss was more evident in the case of osteoporosis with 17 patients (80.9%). This showed that the alveolar bone in patients with osteoarticular diseases such as rheumatoid arthritis and osteoporosis was significantly resorbed, which was of high significance for the study.

**Table 8.** Relationship between tooth mobility and osteoarticular diseases.

| Tooth mobility | Rheumatoid arthritis | | Osteoporosis | | Total | |
|---|---|---|---|---|---|---|
| | No. | % | No. | % | No. | % |
| Grade 1 | 0 | 0,0 | 0 | 0,0 | 0 | 0,0 |
| Grade 2 | 1 | 4,8 | 2 | 9,5 | 3 | 14,3 |
| Grade 3 | 1 | 4,8 | 5 | 23,8 | 6 | 28,6 |
| Grade 4 | 2 | 9,5 | 10 | 47,6 | 12 | 57,1 |
| Total | 4 | 19,1 | 17 | 80,9 | 21 | 100 |

Source: Form

$X^2 = 4{,}184$ $p = 0{,}382$ Not significant

Tooth mobility was present in 21 patients. It was more marked in patients with osteoporosis, occurring in 17 patients (80.9 %) and in the case of rheumatoid arthritis in 4 patients (19.1 %). The prevailing type of mobility was grade 4 with a total of 12 patients (57.1%), followed by grade 3 with 6 patients (28.6%), grade 2 with 3 patients (14.3%) and grade 1 with no patients. It was a clinical sign that was not significant for the study.

**Table 9.** Relationship between real bags and osteoarticular diseases.

| Bags Real | Rheumatoid arthritis | | Osteoporosis | | Total | |
|---|---|---|---|---|---|---|
| | No | % | No | % | No | % |
| 3 mm | 0 | 0,0 | 1 | 4,8 | 1 | 4,8 |
| 4 to 5 mm | 1 | 4,8 | 2 | 9,5 | 3 | 14,3 |
| bowl> 6 mm | 3 | 14,3 | 14 | 66,7 | 17 | 80,9 |
| Total | 4 | 19,1 | 17 | 81 | 21 | 100 |

Source: Form

$X^2 = 8{,}875$ $p = 0{,}003$ Highly Significant

When the actual pockets were measured in the group of pockets greater than or equal to 6 mm, the highest number of patients was found with 17, which accounted for 80.9%. This was followed by the 4 to 5 mm group with 3 patients (14.3%). Pockets measuring 3 mm were found in only 1 patient (4.8%). This showed that the pathological deepening of the gingival sulcus was of great importance as most of the patients had it and its value was of great significance.

**Table 10.** Risk factors associated with chronic periodontal disease and osteoarticular diseases.

| Risk factors | Chronic Periodontal Disease | | | | Diseases Osteoarticular | | | |
|---|---|---|---|---|---|---|---|---|
| | Gingivitis | | Periodontitis | | Osteoporosis | | Rheumatoid arthritis | |
| | No | % | No | % | No | % | No | % |
| PDB | 11 | 34,4 | 21 | 65,6 | 16 | 50,0 | 7 | 21,9 |
| Tobacco | 6 | 18,8 | 12 | 37,5 | 10 | 31,3 | 9 | 28,1 |
| Stress | 11 | 34,4 | 20 | 62,5 | 20 | 62,5 | 12 | 37,5 |
| Immunodeficiencies | 2 | 6,3 | 3 | 9,4 | 10 | 31,3 | 10 | 31,3 |
| Genetics | 10 | 31,3 | 12 | 37,5 | 14 | 43,8 | 8 | 25 |
| Xerostomia | 1 | 3,1 | 8 | 25 | 12 | 37,5 | 10 | 31,3 |
| Harmful habits | 6 | 18,8 | 13 | 40,6 | 2 | 6,3 | 1 | 3,1 |
| Poor Oral Hygiene | 10 | 31,3 | 19 | 59,4 | 14 | 43,8 | 8 | 25 |

Source: Form

The risk factors with the highest incidence of periodontal diseases were the presence of PDB, stress and poor oral hygiene with 11 patients with PDB and stress and 10 with poor oral hygiene for chronic gingivitis, representing 34.4% and 31.3% respectively; with regard to chronic periodontitis these factors also predominated with 21 patients with PDB for 65.6%, stress with 20 patients for 62.5% and poor oral hygiene with 19 patients for 59.4%. With regard to osteoarticular diseases in the case of osteoporosis, stress was more representative with 20 patients representing 62.5 % and the presence of dental plaque with 16 patients representing 50 %. In the case of rheumatoid arthritis it was also stress, but with 12 patients for 37.5%, followed by xerostomia and immunodeficiencies both with 10 patients for 31.3%. These results showed that stress played a major role in both the occurrence of periodontopathies and the development of bone disease.

**Table 11.** Relationship between chronic periodontal disease and osteoporosis.

| Disease<br>Chronic periodontal | Osteoporosis | | | |
|---|---|---|---|---|
| | Yes | | No. | |
| | No. | % | No. | % |
| Chronic gingivitis | 3 | 9,4 | 8 | 25,0 |
| Chronic periodontitis | 17 | 53,1 | 4 | 12,5 |
| Total | 20 | 62,5 | 12 | 37,5 |

Source: Form

X2 = 8.875 p = 0.003 Highly Significant

Chronic periodontitis was the most prevalent periodontal disease in patients with osteoporosis with 17 patients representing 53.1% of the total. Chronic gingivitis had 3 patients for 9.4%. It was observed that osteoporosis and periodontitis, having similar bone destruction patterns, manifested themselves in combination to a greater extent in the patients and their relationship had a high significance in the statistical analysis.

**Table 12.** Relationship between Chronic Periodontal Disease and Rheumatoid Arthritis

| Chronic Periodontal Disease | Rheumatoid arthritis | | | |
|---|---|---|---|---|
| | Yes | | No. | |
| | No. | % | No. | % |
| Chronic gingivitis | 8 | 25,0 | 3 | 9,4 |
| Chronic periodontitis | 4 | 12,5 | 17 | 53,1 |
| Total | 12 | 37,5 | 20 | 62,5 |

Source: Form

$X^2$ = 8,875 p = 0,003 Highly Significant

The most prevalent periodontal disease in relation to rheumatoid arthritis was chronic gingivitis with 8 patients representing 25.0 % of the total. In the case of chronic periodontitis, there were 4 patients who manifested both diseases at the same time, which constituted 12.5% of the total. This showed a stronger link between rheumatoid arthritis and gingivitis. The relationship between these diseases was highly significant.

## Discussion of the results:

It was observed that the age group most affected by chronic periodontal disease and osteoarticular diseases was 61-65 years and the sex was female. These results coincided with those obtained by González Febles[14] in this age group; however, they differ from the results of Soto[53] and Garrido[71] in both sex and age group. Antúnez[58] reported greater affectation in the 35-49 age group, which was similar to the present study, but did not coincide in relation to sex. No statistically significant relationship was found between age and sex. It was also similar to that of Camaño[60] , in whose study the female sex predominated.

According to the author's criteria, between the ages of 51 and 55, women suffer a series of hormonal disorders linked to the menopause, which means that they begin to suffer from oral symptoms typical of this physiological situation. She also notes that, at this stage, in general, new systemic pathologies begin to appear that lead to a lack of concern for oral health.

Loredo[22] stated that the greater affectation in terms of gender could be linked to the fact that the female gender was more susceptible to dental morbidity. Iglesias Estrada[57] reported different results, with the most frequent conditions occurring in men.

Periodontal disease was diagnosed according to clinical characteristics and X-ray findings. Chronic periodontitis predominated and chronic gingivitis was the least represented. The female sex was predominant. According to a study by Heras Barsallo[5] , chronic gingivitis predominated over chronic periodontitis due to the coverage of services which, with timely treatment, prevented the disease from progressing to a higher stage. It was influenced by socio-economic and socio-cultural factors. This was not consistent with this research.

According to the age groups in the sample, the 61-65 years age group predominated. This behaviour showed that this age group was more susceptible to developing chronic periodontal disease. Villegas Rojas[31] reports that, according to age, periodontal disease was more or less frequent, which depended on the characteristics of each patient, but the majority was more frequent in adulthood, which reaffirmed the results obtained in this research.

In the case of osteoarticular diseases, the female sex also predominated and osteoporosis was more prevalent than rheumatoid arthritis. Authors such as Almutairi[15] and Armas[59] agreed with these data in their studies. In the study by Bedoya[62] , the male sex predominated when analysing osteoarticular diseases in workers in the agricultural sector. The present study demonstrated with these data points of coincidence with respect to periodontal disease.

The age of 61 to 65 years was predominant for patients with osteoarticular diseases, as was reported by Pino Falconí[6] 4, who stated: In all cases and as the age of the participants increased, the densitometric values of women with periodontitis were lower than those of women without periodontitis.

The clinical signs of chronic periodontal disease that predominated in relation to osteoarticular diseases were gingivorrhoea, virtual pockets, real pockets, bone loss and tooth mobility. Where gingivorrhoea predominated.

The author Soto-Gil[53] reported an increase in the rate of bleeding and catheterisation in patients with rheumatoid arthritis, although for Dris Hamed[52] there was no such difference in this parameter.

In the literature, the study by author Katz JD[10] found significant differences in attachment loss and periodontal pockets, which were significantly higher in patients with rheumatoid arthritis. In contrast, the analysis by Molon RS[13] found no such difference between patients with rheumatoid arthritis and those without.

Although differences were shown between patients with rheumatoid arthritis with and without periodontal disease the results are not statistically significant as was the case with researcher Ferrer F.[68] in his analysis.

In relation to osteoporosis, a relationship between low bone mass and decreased clinical attachment loss has been reported, as in the case of the scientific study of menopausal women by Fonseca A. [77] which showed that the highest levels of clinical attachment loss were found in those with lower bone density, in addition to significantly greater pocket depth and interproximal alveolar bone loss compared to the non-osteoporotic group, which coincided with the values reported in this study where the presence of real pockets and vertical bone loss were predominant. Also the presence or absence of subgingival plaque was associated with bone mineral density and the amelocemental boundary as reported by Manjunath SH[72] in their research.

He concurred this report with the recent study by author Mongkornkarn S.[73] which showed that patients with reduced oral hygiene and severe periodontitis also had osteoporosis, another study by Ayed MS.[74] concluded that osteoporosis was an important risk factor for periodontal disease and appeared to act as a driver of periodontal disease.

With regard to the risk factors common to the diseases in question, stress and the presence of dentobacterial plaque were relevant, with higher values for both periodontal diseases and osteoarticular diseases. An increased amount of dentobacterial plaque was demonstrated in patients with rheumatoid arthritis compared to patients without the disease as reported by Soto-Gil[53] . Another study, by Cuenca Miño[29] showed that antibody levels were significantly higher in patients with rheumatoid arthritis and advanced periodontal disease than in patients with rheumatoid arthritis without periodontal disease. However, Borja Ibarra K.[75] found no such differences and even observed some improvement in the amount of plaque in patients with rheumatoid arthritis. With respect to stress, it was revealed that it produced a dysregulation of the immune system, through complex interactions with the neuroendocrine axis. In periodontal disease, this factor, in addition to directly altering the immune response, could intervene through unhealthy behaviours, which increased the risk of developing periodontal disease. In many patients, it was observed that the first manifestations and symptomatic flare-ups of rheumatoid arthritis were preceded by periods of stress as found in the studies of Dris Hamed[52] and Guevara 11.

The study proved the link between periodontal disease and osteoporosis, which prevailed in the case of periodontitis. He agreed with the findings of Vizcaino Bautista[16] who argued that there were similarities between the two diseases. Both osteoporosis and periodontal diseases are processes that shared pathogenic mechanisms and were determined by a decrease in bone mass and gradual bone resorption; they presented a prevalence that increased as the population aged. Their progression or severity could lead to local or systemic involvement. They disagreed with the study by Jordan PM[17] which stated that the data were not conclusive enough to establish a strong relationship between the two diseases.

When we then looked at periodontal disease and rheumatoid arthritis, we could see how it was more closely related to gingivitis. Both diseases were characterised by chronic inflammation, soft tissue damage, similar cellular and humoral immune response and a common genetic background. As for the relationship between periodontitis and rheumatoid arthritis, it was given by the significant and constant increase of genetic and inflammatory mediators, as well as microbial endotoxin products, these common characteristics were demonstrated by the author Hernandez Batista[61] in his analysis.

The results obtained during this investigation did not coincide with the study by Rodríguez Lozano et al.[76] where a statistically significant association between periodontitis and rheumatoid arthritis was observed. Compared to controls, patients with rheumatoid arthritis presented worse periodontal status, which was statistically significant. Following ordinal regression modelling, a statistically significant association was observed between periodontitis severity and rheumatoid arthritis activity.

## Conclusions:

The study found that the most affected age group was 61-65, with a higher proportion of women.

A predominance of clinical signs of chronic periodontal disease was observed, with gingivorrhoea being the most prominent, followed by the presence of real pockets, bone loss and tooth mobility in relation to the osteoarticular diseases rheumatoid arthritis and osteoporosis.

The risk factors with the highest incidence of chronic periodontal disease were the presence of PDB and stress.

A relationship between periodontal diseases chronic gingivitis and chronic periodontitis and osteoarticular diseases rheumatoid arthritis and osteoporosis was demonstrated. Patients with osteoporosis were more associated with the occurrence of chronic periodontitis. Those with rheumatoid arthritis were more associated with chronic gingivitis.

## Bibliographical references:


1 Uzho Cabrera AJ. Diabetes mellitus and periodontal disease in young patients [Internet]. Guayaquil: [s.l] 2019.(Cited 2024,Jan 21). Available from: http://repositorio.ug.edu.ec/bitstream/redug/44269/1/UZHOalonso.pdf

2' WHO estimates that oral diseases affect nearly 3.5 billion people [Internet]. Madrid; 2023.(Cited 2023 ,Jun 11) Available from: https://www.infosalus.com/salud-investigacion/noticia))who-estimates-oral-diseases-affect-almost-3500-million-persons-20200320140129.html

3. Mamani Cahuata Balia. Periodontal disease as a risk factor for systemic diseases in Latin America. Bibliographic review. Peru. 2021

4 Bilgin Cetin, M., Sezgin, Y., Nisanci Yilmaz, M. N., & Köseoglu Sezgin, C.. Assessment of carotid artery calcifications on digital panoramic radiographs and their relationship with periodontal condition and cardiovascular risk factors. International Dental Journal.(2020) doi: 10.1111/idj.12618

5. Heras Barsallo MR. Prevalence of periodontal disease in adults in Latin America [Internet]. 2021.(Cited 2024,Feb 16) Available at: https://dspace.ucacue.edu.ec/handle/ucacue/11337

6. Gamonal J, Bravo J, Malheiros Z, Stewart B, Morales A, Cavalla F, Gomez M. Periodontal disease and its impact on general health status in Latin America. Section I: Introduction (part I). Braz Oral Res. 2019; 34(1):e024.

7' González Díaz ME and collective of authors. Compendium of Periodontics. Havana: Editorial Ciencias Médicas; 2017.

8' Morffi Serrano Y. Social and economic impact of periodontopathies in the population. CCM [Internet] 2015 [cited 2023, Apr 12];19(2): [approx. 6 p.]. Available from:

http://scieloprueba.sld.cu/scielo.php?script=sci_arttext&pid=S1560-43812015000200017&lng=es&nrm=iso

9' Hartvigsen J, Hancock MJ, Kongsted A, et al. What low back pain is and why we need to pay attention. Lancet 2018; 391: 2356-67.

10. Katz JD, Walitt B. Rheumatic diseases in older adults. Rheum Dis Clin N Am. 2018 [Accessed 2023, Jun 14]; 44(3): 13-14. Available from: https://doi.org/10.1016/j.rdc.2018.05.001

11 Guevara Acurio Ángela Lissette, Ramos Veintimilla Wendy Yadira, Guevara Leguisano Daniel Asdruval, Pino Falconí Pablo Ernesto. Therapeutic approaches to osteoporosis. Rev Cuba Reumatol [Internet]. 2022 Apr [cited 2024 Feb 16]; 24(1):e237. Available from:

http://scielo.sld.cu/scielo.php?script=sci_arttext&pid=S_1817-_59962022000100012&lng=en. Epub 01-Apr-2022.

12. Cieza, A., Causey, K., Kamenov, K., Hanson, S. W., Chatterji, S., &Vos, T. (2020). Global

estimates of the need for rehabilitation based on the Global Burden of Disease study 2019: a systematic analysis for the Global Burden of Disease Study 2019. The Lancet, 396(10267).

13. de Molon RS, Rossa C Jr, Thurlings RM, Cirelli JA, Koenders MI. Linkage of Periodontitis and Rheumatoid Arthritis: Current Evidence and Potential Biological Interactions. IJMS. 2019 Sep; 20(18): 4541-35.

1 4' González Febles Jerián. Association between the severity of periodontitis and the severity of rheumatoid arthritis. Doctoral thesis. Madrid 2021

15 Almutairi K, Nossent J, Preen D, Keen H, Inderjeeth C. The global prevalence of rheumatoid arthritis: a meta-analysis based on a systematic review. Rheumatol Int. 2nd ed. Springer Berlin Heidelberg; 2020 Nov 11; 6: 468-15.

16 Vizcaino Bautista Estefany Nataly. Periodontal disease and osteoporosis. Degree work. Guayaquil: University of Guayaquil, 2020. Oct

17. Jordán PM, Blanco PME, Saavedra JLM, et al. Osteoporosis, a health problem of our times. Rev Méd Electron. 2021; 43(2): 12 - 16.

18' Ministry of Public Health. Anuario Estadístico de Salud de Cuba 2020. Havana: MINSAP; 2021 [cited 20 Apr 2023]. Available from: https://files.sld.cu/bvscuba/files/2021/08/Anuario-Estadistico-Espa%c3%b1ol- 2020-Definitivo.pdf

19. Sojod B, Périer JM, Zalcberg A, Bouzegza S, El Halabi B, Anagnostou F. Periodontal disease and general health. EMC-Treaty of Medicine [Internet]. 2022 Mar [cited 12 Jul 2023]; 26(1): 1-8.Available from: https://www.sciencedirect.com/science/article/abs/pii/S1636541022460430

20' Pardo Romero Fredy F, Hernández Luis J. Periodontal disease: epidemiological approaches for its analysis as a public health problem. Journal of Public Health. 2018; 20(2): 5-8. Available at: https://doi.org/10.15446/rsap.V20n2.64

21. Acosta Cruz A, Céspedes Alfonso M, Mayán Reina E. Risk factors and chronic immunoinflammatory periodontal disease in the Clínica Estomatológica Ana Betancourt. Rev Apr 16. 2021; 60(259)

22. Loredo Sandoval Yenit, Cruz Morales Rosario, Cazamayor Laime Zuleica, Montero Arguelles Mayra. Behaviour of chronic immunoinflammatory periodontal disease. Jovellanos. Matanzas. Rev. Med. Electrón. [Internet]. 2019 Feb [cited 2024 Jan 25]; 41(1:78-89. Available from: http:// scielo. sld.cu/ scielo.php?script=sci_arttext&pid=S 1684-18242019000100078&lng=en.

23' Muhammad, N., Al-Ansari, A., Khalifa, A.-K., Muhanad, A., Balgis, G., & Khalid, A. Global Prevalence of Periodontal Disease and Lack of Its Surveillance. The scientific World Journal, 2020(Cited 2024, Mar 2); (5) 1-8. Available at: https://doi.org/10.1155/2020/2146160

24' Martinez Martinez C. Alicia, Llerena E. María, Peña Herrera Manosalva S. María. Prevalence of periodontal disease and associated risk factors.

Dom Sci. 2017(Cited 2024, Feb 24); 3(1): 12-16. Available at http://dx.doi.Org/10.23857/dom.cien.pocaip.2017.3.1.99-108

25' Liccardo D, Cannavo A, Spagnuolo G, Ferrara N, Cittadini A, Rengo C, et al. Periodontal Disease: A Risk Factor for Diabetes and Cardiovascular Disease. Int J Mol Sci. 2019[cited 2023, Jun 25]; 20(6): 1414. Available from: https://www.ncbi.nlm.nih.gov/pmc/articles/PMC6470716/pdf/ijms-20-01414.pdf.

[26]Corona Martínez JD, Pérez Soto E, Sánchez Monroy V. Molecular identification of bacteria in periodontal health and disease. Rev Odont Mex. 2019[cited 2023, Jun 25]; 23(1): 23-30. Available from:

http://www.scielo.org.mx/scielo.php?script=sci arttext&pid=S1870-199X2019000100023&lng=es

27. Sánchez Artigas R, Sánchez Sánchez JR, Sigcho Romero CR, Expósito Lara A. Risk factors for periodontal disease. Correo Científico Médico (CCM) 2021; 25(1): 25-36.

28' Martínez Pérez ML, Camejo Roviralta L, Sánchez Sánchez RJ. Relationship between periodontal disease and ischaemic heart disease. CCM. 2019 [cited 2023, Aug 16]; 23(4): [approx. 6 p]. Available from:

http://www.revcocmed.sld.cu/index.php/cocmed/article/view/3345

29 Cuenca Miño Daniel Humberto. Risk factors related to periodontal disease. Peru: University of Guayaquil; Oct 2020.

30' de la Hoz Rojas Liset, Sarduy Bermúdez Lázaro, Daniel Saura Jesús, Pérez de la Hoz Ana Beatriz, Ruiz Rodríguez Ernesto Luis, Ramos Morales Ana Laura. Patogenio Web en Periodoncia. Villa Clara: University of Medical Sciences; 2020.

31 Villegas Rojas Ivernis Mercedes, Díaz Rivero Abdiel, Domínguez Fernández Yodenis, Solís Cabrera Berta Alina, Tabares Alonso Yadelis. Prevalence and severity of periodontal disease in diabetic patients. Rev. Med. Electron [Internet]. 2018 Dec [cited 2024 Jan 25]: 40(6): 1911-30. Available

http://scielo.sld.cu/scielo.php?script=sci_arttext&pid=S1684- 18242018000601911&lng=es.

32. Zhang Y, He J, He B, Huang R, Li M. Effect of tobacco on periodontal disease and oral cancer. Tob Induc Dis. 2019[cited 2023 Jan 14]; 17:40. Available from: https://doi.org/10.18332/tid/106187

33' Pardo Romero, F. F., & Hernández, L. J. Periodontal disease: Epidemiological approaches for its analysis as a public health problem. Journal of Public Health. 2018(Cited 2024, Jun 24); 20:258-64. Available at: https://doi.org/10.15446/rsap.v20n2.64654

34' Bombino, L. P., Pimentel, B. F. T., & Cabarrocas, F. V. Chronic inflammatory periodontal disease and cardiovascular disease. Guayaquil; 2020. p 23.

35. López Tovar GP. Epidemiology of periodontal disease. Peru: University of Guayaquil; 2021 Sep.

36. Ko, T.-J., Byrd, K., & Kim, S. The Chairside Periodontal Diagnostic Toolkit: Past, Present, and future. Diagnostics. 2021(Cited 2024, Feb 16); 11(6): 1-23. doi: https://doi.org/10.3390/diagnostics11060932

37. Herrera David, Figuero Elena, Lior Shapira, Jin Lijian, Sanz Mariano.The new classification of periodontal and peri-implant diseases.Revista Científica de la Sociedad Española de Periodoncia. 2018; 11(5): p14.

38. Albandar JM, Susin C, Hughes FJ. Manifestations of systemic diseases and conditions that affect the periodontal attachment apparatus: Case definitions and diagnostic considerations. Journal of Clinical Periodontology. 2018; 45, S89- S171.

39 Araujo M, Lindhe J. Peri-implant health. Journal of Clinical Periodontology (2018)45; S230-S236.

40. Berglundh T, Armitage GC, Ávila-Ortiz G et al. Consensus Report: Peri-implant Diseases and Conditions. Journal of Clinical Periodontology (2018)45, S286-S291.

41 Chapple ILC, Mealey BL, van Dyke TE et al. Consensus report: Periodontal health and gingival diseases/conditions. Journal of Clinical Periodontology (2018) 45, S68-S77.

42. Lang NP, Bartold PM. Periodontal health. Journal of Clinical Periodontology (2018) 45, S9-S16.

43. Cárdenas-Valenzuela Paola, Guzmán-Gastelum Dalia Abril, Valera-González Eligio, Cuevas-González Juan Carlos, Zambrano-Galván Graciela, García- Calderón Alma Graciela. Main Diagnostic Criteria of the New Classification of Periodontal Diseases and Conditions. Int. J. Odontostomat. [Internet]. 2021 Mar [cited 2024 Feb 07]; 15(1): 175-80. Available from: http://www.scielo.cl/scielo.php?script=sci arttext&pid=S0718-381X2021000100175&lng=en.http://dx.doi.org/10.4067/S0718-381X2021000100175

44 Graetz, C.; Mann, L.; Krois, J.; Sälzer, S.; Kahl M.; Springer, C. & Schwendicke, F. Comparison of periodontitis patients' classification in the 2018 versus 1999 classification. J. Clin. Periodontol. 2019,46(9):908-17.

45. Dietrich, T.; Ower, P.; Tank, M.; West, N. X.; Walter, C.; Needleman, I.; Hughes, F. J.; Wadia, R.; Milward, M. R.; Hodge, P. J.; et al. Periodontal diagnosis in the context of the 2017 classification system of periodontal diseases and conditions - implementation in clinical practice. Br. Dent. J.2019; 226(1):16-22.

46. Zerón Agustín. The new classification of periodontal diseases. ADM Journal.2018 May Jun,LXXV(3)

47. Gutiérrez-Romero Fabiola, Padilla-Avalos César Augusto, Marroquín-Soto Consuelo. Periodontal disease in Latin America: regional approach and health strategy. Rev. Public Health [Internet]. August 2022 [accessed February 7, 2024]; 24(4):6-10. Available at: http://www.scielo.org.co/scielo.php?script=sci_arttext&pid=S0124-00642022000400130&lng=en.

48' Peres MA, Macpherson LMD, Weyant RJ, Daly B, Venturelli R, Mathur MR, et al. Oral diseases: a global public health challenge. Lancet. 2019; 394(10194):249-60. Disponible en: https://doi.org/10.1016/s0140-6736(19)31146-8.

49 López Sandoval MB. Management of antibiotic therapy in periodontal disease. Peru: University of Guayaquil; 2019 Sep.

50' Palenzuela-Ramos Y, Moreira-Díaz LR, Padrón-Álvarez JE. Osteogenesis imperfecta, report of a case. Place of publication: Universidad Médica Pinareña. 2020; 16(2):1-6.

51 Valdéz Mérito Rafael Moisés. Osteoarticular_Pathologies. Class 19. 2018

52. Dris Hamed AF. Association between periodontal disease and rheumatoid arthritis [thesis]. Seville: University of Seville; 2020 [cited 2023, Jul 28]. Available from:https://idus.us.es/bitstream/handle/11441/104470/Asociaci%c3%b3n%20entre%20la%20enfermedad%20periodontal%20y%20la%20artritis%20reumatoide.pdf?sequence=1&isAllowed=y

53. Soto-Gil Marileivy, Gil-Figueroa Bertha Vivian, Careaga-Valido Dianelys.

Manifestations of periodontal disease in patients with rheumatoid arthritis. Arch Méd Camagüey [Internet]. 2023 [cited 2024 Feb 07]; 27:e9452. Available from:

http:// scielo. sld.cu/ scielo.php?script=sci_arttext&pid=S 1025-02552023000100029&lng=en. Epub 25-Apr-2023.

54' Kamer AR, Craig RG, Niederman R, Fortea J, de Leon MJ. Periodontal disease as a possible cause for Alzheimer's disease. Periodontol 2000. John Wiley & Sons, Ltd; 2020 Jun; 83(1):242-71.

55' Sanz M, Marco del Castillo A, Jepsen S, González Juanatey JR, D'Aiuto F, Bouchard P, et al. Periodontitis and cardiovascular diseases: Consensus report. J Clin Periodontol. 2020 Feb 3; 311(14):e318-21.

56' Figuero E, Han YW, Furuichi Y. Periodontal diseases and adverse pregnancy outcomes: Mechanisms. Periodontol 2000. John Wiley & Sons, Ltd; 2020 Jun; 83(1):175-88.

57 Iglesias Estrada YH, Viamontes Beltrán J, Rodríguez Caballero RR, Mazorra Rivera A. Manifestations of periodontal disease in patients with rheumatoid arthritis. Revista Progaleno [Internet]. 2018 [cited 2023, Jul 12]; 1(2). Available from:https://revprogaleno.sld.cu/index.php/progaleno/article/view/18/13

58' Antúnez Fernández FI. Periodontal disease and its relationship with systemic diseases [thesis]. Xochimilco: Universidad Autónoma Metropolitana; 2021 [cited 2023, Jul 12]. Available from: Available from: https://repositorio.xoc.uam.mx/jspui/bitstream/123456789/26229/1/cbsCD130422163310ypap.pdf.

59. Armas Rodríguez WE, Alarcón Medina GA, Ocampo Dávila FD, Arteaga CM,

Arteaga Paredes PA. Rheumatoid arthritis, diagnosis, evolution and treatment. Rev cuban rheumatol [Internet]. 2019 [cited 2023, Jul 12]; 21(3):[approx. p7]. Available from: Available from: https://revreumatologia.sld.cu/index.php/reumatologia/article/view/759/html

60. Camaño Carballo L, Pimienta Concepción I. Oral involvement in patients with rheumatoid arthritis. Rev cuban rheumatol [Internet]. 2020 [cited 2023, Jul 12]; 22(2). Available from: Available from: https://revreumatologia.sld.cu/index.php/reumatologia/article/view/783/1475

61' Hernández Batista SC, Villafuerte Morales JE, Chimbolema Mullo SO, Pilamunga Lema CL. Cardiovascular risk factors in patients with rheumatic diseases. Rev cuban rheumatol [Internet]. 2020 Apr [cited 2023, Jul 28]; 22(1). Available from: Available from: https://revreumatologia.sld.cu/index.php/reumatologia/article/view/723/1434

62' Bedoya Narvaez Daniela, Fernández Aragón Laura V. Relation of musculoskeletal and osteoarticular diseases with exposure to biomechanical hazard in workers in the agricultural sector worldwide in the last eight years. Institución Universitaria Antonio José.Santiago de Cali.2020.

63. Acosta Cruz A, Céspedes Alfonso M, Mayán Reina G. Risk factors and chronic immunoinflammatory periodontal disease in the Clínica Estomatológica Ana Betancourt. April 16 [Internet]. 2021 [cited 2023, Jul 16]; 60(259):e1085. Available from: https://www.medigraphic.com/pdfs/abril/abr-2021/abr21279h.pdf

64' Pino Falconí PE, Moya Romero KS, Ramos Veintimilla WY, Guevara Acurio AL. Pathogenesis of rheumatoid arthritis, current therapeutic management and future perspectives. Rev cuban rheumatol [Internet]. 2021 Sep-Dec [cited 2023, Jul 16]; 23(3):3-6. Available from: http:// scielo. sld.cu/ scielo.php?script=sci_arttext&pid=S 1817599620210003000 10

65' Rodríguez-Montaño R, Aguilar-Carrillo JA, Bernard-Medina AG, Martínez- Rodríguez VMC, Gómez-Meda BC, Guerrero-Velázquez C. Relationship of periodontitis and rheumatoid arthritis through the IL-23/IL-17a axis. Rev Mex Periodontol [Internet]. 2019 [cited 2023, Jul 28]; X (3):69-76. Available from: https://www.medigraphic.com/pdfs/periodontologia/mp-2019/mp193g.pdf

66. Durán Garnica O, Martínez Sandoval G, Rodríguez Pulido J, Chapa G, Enríquez M. Association of rheumatoid arthritis and periodontitis. Odontología Actual [Internet]. 2020 Dec [cited 2023, Jul 28]; 17(212):28-34. Available from: https://doi.org/10.2307/j.ctv103xbr4.5

67. Peña Cardelles JF, Ortega Concepción D, Cano Durán JA, Melero Alarcón C, Sánchez Labrador Martínez L, De Arriba de la Fuente L, et al. Oral manifestations related to rheumatoid arthritis. Cient Dent [Internet]. 2019 [cited 2023, Jul 12] ;(16)1:73-6. Available from:https://coem.org.es/pdf/publicaciones/cientifica/vol16num1/ArtritisReumatoi de.pdf

68' Ferrer F, Lugo G. Clinical periodontal parameters in patients with a diagnosis of rheumatoid arthritis attending the rheumatology service of the Hospital Clínico Universitario. Case series. Odous Científica [Internet]. 2019 Jul-Dec [cited 2023, Jul 15]; 20(2): 147-164. Available from: http://servicio.bc.uc.edu.ve/odontologia/revista/vol20n2/art06.pdf

69. Cordoví Jiménez A, Díaz Valdés L, Valle Lizama RL, Pérez García LM. Chronic immunoinflammatory periodontal disease and risk factors in adolescents from sports institutions. Gac Méd Espirit [Internet]. 2021 Sep-Dec [cited 2023, Jul 15]; 23(3):74-83. Available from: http://scielo.sld.cu/scielo.php?script=sci arttext&pid=S1608-89212021000300074&lng=en

70' Valarezo Farias SI. Relationship of periodontal pathogens with systemic diseases [thesis]. Guayaquil: Universidad de Guayaquil; 2021 [cited 2023, Jul 15 ] Available from: http://repositorio.ug.edu.ec/bitstream/redug/56077/1/3967VALAREZOsalomon. pdf

71 Garrido Martínez M. Relationship between Periodontal Disease and Osteoporosis. Granada: University of Granada. Doctoral thesis. 2016-2019. Available at: http:handle.net.

72' Manjunath SH, Rakhewar P, Nahar P, Tambe V, Gabhane M, Kharde A. Evaluation of the Prevalence and Severity of Periodontal Diseases between Osteoporotic and Nonosteoporotic Subject: A Cross sectional Comparative Study. The journal of contemporary dental practice. 2019 Oct 1; 20(10):1223_8.

73' Mongkornkarn s, Suthasinekul R, Sritara C, Lertpimonchai A, Tamsailom S,

Udomsak A. Significant association between skeletal bone mineral density and moderate to severe periodontitis in fair oral hygiene individuals. Journal of investigative and clinical dentistry. 2019 Nov 1;10(4):e12441

74' Ayed MS, Alsharif AF, Divakar DD, Jhugroo C, Alosaimi B, Mustafa M. Evaluating the possible association between systemic osteoporosis and periodontal disease progression in postmenopausal women. Disease a Month.2019 Jun1, 6586:193-215.

75. Borja Ibarra. Risk factors for periodontal diseases.Universidad de Guayaquil.2021 Oct 26.

76. Rodríguez-Lozano Beatriz et al. Association between periodontitis severity and clinical disease activity in patients with rheumatoid arthritis: a case-control study. 2019(Cited 2024, Feb 16); 21:27. Available at: https://doi.org/10.1186/s13075-019-1808-z Fonseca, A., & Rueda, R. Effectiveness of hormone replacement therapy as an adjuvant in the treatment of periodontitis in patients with osteoporosis. ODOUS CIENTIFICA, 2019(Cited 2024, Feb 16); (3):97-108.

**Annex 2:**

**Form:**

Name and surname:

Age:

Sex: ___ F ____ M

HEA:

---

Bone pathologies present:

_Rheumatoid arthritis ____ Osteoporosis

Immunodeficiency pathologies: _ Yes _No

Family history of chronic periodontal disease: Yes _No

Stress: _Yes _No

Habits present:

Toothbrushing, times per day: __ 1 __ 2 __ 3 ___4 __ None.

Smoker: ___ Yes _ No

Chewing:_____ Unilateral ____ Bilateral

Signs and symptoms of chronic periodontal disease:

Bleeding on brushing

Bleeding to the borehole

Oedematous gums

Partial loss of stippling

Loss of marginal or papillary morphology

Tooth mobility

Periodontal recession

Periodontal pockets:

_ Real: _3 mm _4 to 5 mm _bol> 6 mm

_ Virtual

Halitosis

Bone losses: _ Horizontal _ Vertical

Dentobacterial Plaque

Xerostomia

Periodontal diagnosis:

Chronic gingivitis

Chronic periodontitis

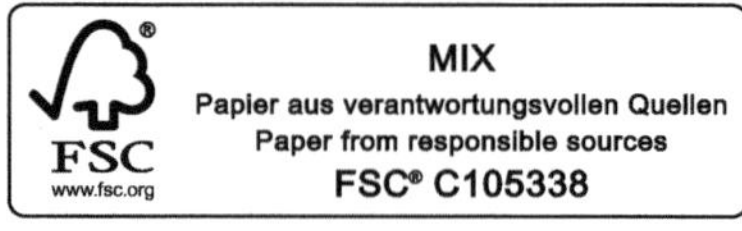


Printed by Books on Demand GmbH, Norderstedt / Germany